The challenge of obesity in the WHO European Region and the strategies for response

Summary

Printing of this publication was supported by the Ministry of Social Affairs and Health of Finland.

The World Health Organization was established in 1948 as the specialized agency of the United Nations responsible for directing and coordinating authority for international health matters and public health. One of WHO's constitutional functions is to provide objective and reliable information and advice in the field of human health. It fulfils this responsibility in part through its publications programmes, seeking to help countries make policies that benefit public health and address their most pressing public health concerns.

The WHO Regional Office for Europe is one of six regional offices throughout the world, each with its own programme geared to the particular health problems of the countries it serves. The European Region embraces some 880 million people living in an area stretching from the Arctic Ocean in the north and the Mediterranean Sea in the south and from the Atlantic Ocean in the west to the Pacific Ocean in the east. The European programme of WHO supports all countries in the Region in developing and sustaining their own health policies, systems and programmes; preventing and overcoming threats to health; preparing for future health challenges; and advocating and implementing public health activities.

To ensure the widest possible availability of authoritative information and guidance on health matters, WHO secures broad international distribution of its publications and encourages their translation and adaptation. By helping to promote and protect health and prevent and control disease, WHO's books contribute to achieving the Organization's principal objective – the attainment by all people of the highest possible level of health.

EUROPE

The challenge of obesity in the WHO European Region and the strategies for response

Summary

Edited by:

Francesco Branca, Haik Nikogosian *and* Tim Lobstein

WHO Library Cataloguing in Publication Data

The challenge of obesity in the WHO European Region and the strategies for response: summary /edited by Francesco Branca, Haik Nikogosian and Tim Lobstein

1.Obesity – prevention and control 2.Obesity – etiology 3.Strategic planning 4.Program development 5.Health policy 6.Europe I.Branca, Francesco II.Nikogosian, Haik III. Lobstein, Tim

ISBN 978 92 890 1388 8 (NLM Classification : WD 210)

ISBN 978 92 890 1388 8

Address requests about publications of the WHO Regional Office for Europe to:

Publications
WHO Regional Office for Europe
Scherfigsvej 8
DK-2100 Copenhagen Ø, Denmark

Alternatively, complete an online request form for documentation, health information, or for permission to quote or translate, on the Regional Office web site (http://www.euro.who.int/pubrequest).

Printed in Denmark

CONTENTS

Acknowledgements vii

Contributors viii

Foreword xi

Executive summary xiii

1. **The challenge** 1
   - Main messages 1
   - Definitions 1
   - Introduction 1
   - Prevalence 2
   - Trends over time 2
   - Intergenerational influences 6
   - Public health effects 8
   - Economic consequences 10
   - Socioeconomic variation in prevalence 10
   - Assessing the challenge: the next steps 12

2. **The determinants of obesity** 13
   - Main messages 13
   - Introduction 13
   - Sedentary behaviour, physical activity, fitness and obesity 14
   - Determinants of physical activity 15
   - Dietary influences on obesity 16
   - Dietary habits in Europe and their relation to obesity 17
   - The food environment 17
   - What drives the food environment 20
   - Food marketing and advertising 21
   - Socioeconomic drivers of obesity 22
   - Obesity and mental health 23
   - Studying the determinants: the next steps 23

3. **The evidence base for interventions to counteract obesity** 24
   - Main messages 24
   - Introduction 24
   - Interventions in micro-settings 25
   - Interventions in macro-settings 27
   - Promoting physical activity 28
   - Economic instruments 28

Considering the context 28
Beyond the experimental evidence 29
Building evidence for effective interventions: the next steps 29

4. Management and treatment of obesity 32
Main messages 32
Introduction 32
Intervention approaches: adults 32
Intervention approaches: children and adolescents 34
Management and treatment: the next steps 35

5. Development of policies to counteract obesity 36
Main messages 36
Introduction 37
Existing international action frameworks 37
Current national policies on obesity in countries of the European Region 39
Development of strategies and action plans 41
An investment approach to health promotion 42
Core actions 43
The role of stakeholders 45
Evaluating policy 46
Policy development: the next steps 47

References 49

Annex 1. European Charter on Counteracting Obesity 56

Acknowledgements

We are grateful to W. Philip T. James (International Obesity Task Force, London, United Kingdom) and Kaare R. Norum (University of Oslo, Norway) for reviews of and suggestions on early drafts of this book, Shubhada Watson (Evidence on Health Needs, WHO Regional Office for Europe) for helping to assess the evidence base, and to Garden Tabacchi (University of Palermo, Italy) for overall editorial assistance in completing the final manuscript.

We also thank the reviewers of the technical content of the papers whose messages are summarized here: Jonathan Back (Directorate-General for Health and Consumer Protection, European Commission, Brussels, Belgium), Leena Eklund (Health Evidence Network, WHO Regional Office for Europe), Egon Jonsson (University of Alberta, Canada), Brian Martin (Federal Office for Sport, Magglingen, Switzerland), Wilfried Kamphausen (Directorate-General for Health and Consumer Protection, European Commission, Luxembourg), Bente Klarlund Pedersen (National University Hospital, Copenhagen, Denmark), Mark Pettigrew (Glasgow, United Kingdom), Claudio Politi (Health Systems Financing, WHO Regional Office for Europe), Pekka Puska, (National Public Health Institute, Helsinki, Finland) and Antonia Trichopoulou (WHO Collaborating Centre for Nutrition Education, University of Athens Medical School, Greece). Useful contributions were also made by Jill Farrington (Noncommunicable Diseases, WHO Regional Office for Europe), Eva Jané-Llopis (Mental Health Promotion and Medical Disorder Prevention, WHO Regional Office for Europe) and Matthijs Muijen (Mental Health, WHO Regional Office for Europe).

Finally, we would like to acknowledge the professional work of the publishing team and the secretarial and communication staff at the WHO Regional Office for Europe, who supported the WHO European Ministerial Conference on Counteracting Obesity and helped make its publications a reality.

Francesco Branca, Haik Nikogosian and Tim Lobstein

Contributors

Ayodola Anise
The Lewin Group, Falls Church, Virginia, United States of America

Tim Armstrong
Chronic Diseases and Health Promotion, WHO headquarters

Colin Bell
Deakin University, Geelong, Australia

Wanda Bemelman
National Institute for Public Health and the Environment, Bilthoven, Netherlands

Vassiliki Benetou
School of Medicine, National and Kapodistrian University of Athens, Athens, Greece

Finn Berggren
Gerlev Physical Education and Sports Academy, Slagelse, Denmark

Lena Björck
Swedish National Food Administration, Uppsala, Sweden

Roar Blom
Noncommunicable Diseases and Lifestyles, WHO Regional Office for Europe

Hendriek Boshuizen
National Institute for Public Health and the Environment, Bilthoven, Netherlands

Francesco Branca
Nutrition and Food Security, WHO Regional Office for Europe

Vanessa Candeias
Chronic Diseases and Health Promotion, WHO headquarters

Margherita Caroli
Prevention Department, Azienda Sanitaria Locale (ASL) Brindisi, Italy

Rob Carter
Health Economics, Deakin University, Melbourne, Australia

Kath Dalmeny
International Association of Consumer Food Organizations, The Food Commission, London, United Kingdom

Mikael Fogelholm
Urho Kekonnen (UKK) Institute for Health Promotion Research, Tampere, Finland

Clifford Goodman
The Lewin Group, Falls Church, Virginia, United States of America

Filippa von Haartman
Swedish National Institute of Public Health, Stockholm, Sweden

Michelle Haby
Department of Human Services, State Government of Victoria, Melbourne, Australia

Richard Heijink
National Institute for Public Health and the Environment, Bilthoven, Netherlands
Rudolf Hoogenveen
National Institute for Public Health and the Environment, Bilthoven, Netherlands
Alan A. Jackson
University of Southampton, United Kingdom
Susan A. Jebb
Elsie Widdowson Laboratory, Cambridge, United Kingdom
Sonja Kahlmeier
Transport and Health, WHO Regional Office for Europe
Ingrid Keller
Noncommunicable Diseases and Mental Health, WHO headquarters
Cécile Knai
London School of Hygiene and Tropical Medicine, United Kingdom
Peter Kopelman
University of East Anglia, Norwich, United Kingdom
Tim Lobstein
International Obesity Task Force, International Association for the Study of Obesity, London, United Kingdom
Brian Martin
Federal Office for Sport, Magglingen, Switzerland
Marjory Moodie
Deakin University, Melbourne, Australia
Androniki Naska
School of Medicine, National and Kapodistrian University of Athens, Greece
Haik Nikogosian
Division of Health Programmes, WHO Regional Office for Europe
Chizuru Nishida
Nutrition for Health and Development, WHO headquarters
Marga C. Ocké
National Institute for Public Health and the Environment, Bilthoven, Netherlands
Pekka Oja
Karolinska Institute, Huddinge, Sweden
Jean-Michel Oppert
Université Pierre et Marie Curie, Paris, France
Johan Polder
National Institute for Public Health and the Environment, Bilthoven, Netherlands
Joceline Pomerleau
London School of Hygiene and Tropical Medicine, United Kingdom
Francesca Racioppi
Transport and Health, WHO Regional Office for Europe

Neville Rigby
International Obesity TaskForce, International Association for the Study of Obesity, London, United Kingdom
Nathalie Röbbel
Environment and Health Coordination and Partnership, WHO Regional Office for Europe
Harry Rutter
South East Public Health Observatory, Oxford, United Kingdom
Liselotte Schäfer Elinder
Swedish National Institute of Public Health, Stockholm, Sweden
Jaap C. Seidell
Free University of Amsterdam, Netherlands
Anne Simmons
Deakin University, Geelong, Australia
Michael Sjöström
Karolinska Institute, Huddinge, Sweden
Annica Sohlström
Swedish National Food Administration, Uppsala, Sweden
Marc Suhrcke
Investment for Health and Development, WHO Regional Office for Europe
Carolyn Summerbell
School of Health and Social Care, University of Teesside, Middlesbrough, United Kingdom
Boyd Swinburn
WHO Collaborating Centre for Obesity Prevention, Deakin University, Melbourne, Australia
Ursula Trübswasser
Nutrition and Food Security, WHO Regional Office for Europe
Agis Tsouros
Healthy Cities and Urban Governance, WHO Regional Office for Europe
Colin Tukuitonga
Noncommunicable Diseases and Mental Health, WHO headquarters
Nienke Veerbeek
Amstelveen, Netherlands
Tommy L.S. Visscher
Free University of Amsterdam, Netherlands
Patricia M.C.M. Waijers
National Institute for Public Health and the Environment, Bilthoven, Netherlands
Trudy M.A. Wijnhoven
Nutrition and Food Security, WHO Regional Office for Europe
Stephen A. Wootton
University of Southampton, United Kingdom
Laura Wyness
Turriff, Scotland, United Kingdom
Agneta Yngve
Karolinska Institute, Huddinge, Sweden

Foreword

In response to the emerging challenge of the obesity epidemic, the WHO Regional Office for Europe organized the WHO European Ministerial Conference on Counteracting Obesity, which took place in Istanbul, Turkey on 15–18 November 2006.

This book is the main background document prepared for the Conference and distils the concepts and conclusions of many papers that were written by a large group of experts in public health, nutrition and medicine and are being published by the Regional Office. Both the summary and the larger book illustrate the dynamics of the epidemic and its impact on public health throughout the WHO European Region. In particular, the obesity epidemic's rapid expansion to the countries in the eastern part of the Region causes great concern, as they now suffer from a double burden of disease linked to both under- and overnutrition.

The epidemic's rapid growth is linked to the global increase in the availability and accessibility of food and the reduced opportunities to use physical energy. Food has never been so affordable, and products high in fats and sugar are the cheapest. Thus, modern societies are seen as "obesogenic" environments: meaning that they lead to overconsumption of food and to widespread sedentary lifestyles, which increase the risk of obesity. The two Conference publications describe how these influences are shaped in different settings, such as the family, school, community and workplace.

The books make both ethical and economic arguments for accelerating action against obesity. In addition to harming the health and well-being of a vast proportion of the population and generating large expenditures by health services, obesity has a striking and unacceptable impact on children. Obese children suffer longer years of exposure to the metabolic syndrome and show health effects such as diabetes earlier in life. Children's obesity is the clearest demonstration of the strength of environmental influences and the failure of the traditional prevention strategies based only on health promotion; children are far more receptive to commercial messages than recommendations from their teachers or health care providers. In addition, policy-makers should note that obesity both results from and causes social gaps. Socially vulnerable groups are more affected by obesity because they live in neighbourhoods that do not facilitate active transport and leisure, they have less access to education and information about lifestyles and health, and cheaper food options are nutrient poor and energy dense.

It is time to act. In Istanbul, the Region's Member States approved the European Charter on Counteracting Obesity (Annex 1), which lists guiding principles and clear action areas. Action should span government sectors, be international and involve multiple stakeholders. The Conference publications analyse effective programmes and policies in different sectors, such as education, health, agriculture and trade, urban planning and transport. They also describe how to design policies and programmes to prevent obesity and how to monitor progress. As to action from stakeholders, they call, for example, on the private sector – including food manufacturers, advertisers and traders – to revise its policies, both voluntarily and as a result of legislation. Professional organizations need to support the prevention and management of obesity and its associated morbidity. Consumers' organizations should collaborate in providing information and in keeping public awareness high. Intergovernmental actors need to ensure that the agreed action is enforced across national borders, by issuing adequate directives and policy guidance.

WHO's role is to provide policy advice based on evidence, to disseminate examples of best practice, to promote political commitment and to lead international action. At the global level, the Global Strategy on Diet, Physical Activity and Health provides clear direction. In the European Region, the First Action Plan for Food and Nutrition Policy placed nutrition on governments' agendas. WHO is now committed to proposing further detailed guidelines in support of this public health priority.

Authoritative observers around the world have received the European Charter on Counteracting Obesity as a useful step forward, owing to its guiding principles and clear directions, and the wide consensus that it represents. This helps to create the right conditions in which countries can halt the increase in childhood obesity and curb overall the epidemic in no more than a decade. We at WHO are working to help make this goal achievable and, indeed, inevitable.

Marc Danzon
WHO Regional Director for Europe

Executive summary

Obesity presents Europe with an unprecedented public health challenge that has been underestimated, poorly assessed and not fully accepted as a strategic governmental problem with substantial economic implications. The epidemic now emerging in children will markedly accentuate the burden of ill health unless urgent steps with novel approaches are taken based on a clear understanding of the economic drivers of the epidemic and a rejection of the traditional everyday assumptions about its causes. Most adults in Europe have poor, inappropriate diets and are physically inactive. The challenge is to avoid the search for a single solution and to develop a coherent, progressive, cross-government and international strategy, based on short-, medium- and long-term societal changes.

Poor diet, a lack of physical activity and the resulting obesity and its associated illnesses are together responsible for as much ill health and premature death as tobacco smoking. Overweight affects between 30% and 80% of adults in the WHO European Region and up to one third of children.

The rates of obesity are rising in virtually all parts of the Region. The costs to the health services of treating the resulting ill health – such as type 2 diabetes, certain types of cancer and cardiovascular diseases – are estimated to be up to 6% of total health care expenditure, and indirect costs in lost productivity add as much again.

The rise in childhood obesity is perhaps even more alarming. Over 60% of children who are overweight before puberty will be overweight in early adulthood, reducing the average age at which noncommunicable diseases become apparent and greatly increasing the burden on health services, which have to provide treatment during much of their adult lives.

Preventing obesity is thus an urgent public health goal that should be dealt with through innovative environmental approaches, very much like the introduction of clean water supplies, sewerage treatment facilities and food inspection services in the 18th and 19th centuries and the recently established controls on air pollution, drink–driving, seat-belt use and smoking in public places.

This publication summarizes a series of research papers commissioned by the WHO Regional Office for Europe as a contribution to the WHO European Ministerial Conference on Counteracting Obesity in Istanbul, Turkey in November 2006, which itself is part of the process of implementing the Global Strategy on Diet, Physical Activity and Health agreed at the World Health Assembly in May 2004 (resolution WHA57.17), the European Strategy for the Prevention and Control of Noncommunicable Diseases (endorsed by the WHO Regional Committee for Europe at its fifty-sixth session in 2006) and the Global Strategy on Infant and Young Child Feeding agreed at the World Health Assembly in May 2002 (resolution WHA55.25). The Regional Office will publish the research papers later this year.

This publication outlines the extent of the problem, the implications for the health sector and other sectors, and the range of interventions needed to halt the rising trend and eventually reverse it. It also outlines national and regional policies for population-level health promotion and disease prevention, action targeting high-risk individuals, and effective treatment and care of obese individuals.

1. The challenge

Main messages

- Overweight and obesity are a serious public health challenge in the WHO European Region.
- The prevalence of obesity is rising rapidly and is expected to include 150 million adults and 15 million children by 2010.
- The obesity trend is especially alarming in children and adolescents. The annual rate of increase in the prevalence of childhood obesity has been growing steadily, and the current rate is 10 times higher than it was in the 1970s. This reinforces the adult epidemic and creates a growing health challenge for the next generation.
- Overweight and obesity are responsible for about 80% of cases of type 2 diabetes, 35% of ischaemic heart disease and 55% of hypertensive disease among adults in the Region and cause more than 1 million deaths and 12 million life-years of ill health each year.
- Obesity is responsible for up to 6% of national health care costs in the WHO European Region.
- Obesity and its associated diseases impair economic development and limit individual economic opportunities.
- Obesity affects the poor in Europe more severely, imposes a larger disease burden on them and handicaps their opportunities for improving their socioeconomic status.

Definitions

In adults, excess body weight is defined as having a body mass index (BMI) ≥25 kg/m^2. Obesity is defined as a BMI ≥30 kg/m^2; pre-obese is used to define adults with a BMI of 25.0–29.9 kg/m^2. In this publication the term overweight means adults with a BMI ≥25 kg/m^2, although some authors mean solely those with a BMI of 25.0–29.9 kg/m^2 *(1)*.

For children and adolescents, there are various different approaches to defining overweight and obesity *(2)*. This publication uses the definition based on the percentile values of BMI adjusted for age and gender that correspond to BMI of 25 and 30 kg/m^2 at age 18 years *(3)*. Prevalence data for children younger than five years may need to be recalculated based on the new WHO Child Growth Standards *(4)*.

Introduction

Excess body weight poses one of the most serious public health challenges of the 21st century for the WHO European Region, where the prevalence of obesity has tripled in the last two decades and has now reached epidemic proportions. If no action is taken and the prevalence of obesity continues to increase at the same rate as in the 1990s, an estimated 150 million adults *(5)* and 15 million children and adolescents *(6)* in the Region will be obese by 2010.

Overweight is responsible for a large proportion of the total burden of disease in the WHO European Region. It is responsible for more than 1 million deaths and 12 million life-years of ill health in the Region every year *(7)*. More than three quarters of the cases of type 2 diabetes are attributable to BMI exceeding 21 kg/m^2; overweight is also a risk factor for ischaemic heart disease, hypertensive disease, ischaemic stroke, colon cancer, breast cancer, endometrial cancer and osteoarthritis. Obesity negatively affects psychosocial health and personal quality of life.

Overweight also affects economic and social development through increased health care costs and loss of productivity and income. Adult obesity is already responsible for up to 6% of the health care expenses in the Region.

The prevalence of obesity varies widely between countries and between different socioeconomic groups within countries, and this highlights the importance of environmental and socio-cultural determinants of diet and physical activity.

Prevalence

Data sets from national and regional studies on the prevalence of overweight and obesity among children, adolescents and adults have been compiled from existing databases, published literature, scientists and health agencies. Information on the current situation (data collected in the past six years) is now available for 46 of 52 countries in the WHO European Region.[1] Local data have been used in the absence of nationally representative figures.

Adults

In countries that have carried out measurements, the prevalence of overweight ranged between 32% and 79% in men and between 28% and 78% in women. The highest prevalence was found in Albania (in Tirana), Bosnia and Herzegovina and the United Kingdom (in Scotland); Turkmenistan and Uzbekistan had the lowest rates. The prevalence of obesity ranged from 5% to 23% among men and between 7% and 36% among women. Self-reported data generally underestimate the prevalence of obesity, especially among overweight women. The prevalence obtained from self-reports can be up to 50% lower than the prevalence calculated from weight and height measurements.

The prevalence of obesity was higher among men than among women in 14 of 36 countries or regions with data for both genders, whereas the prevalence of pre-obesity was higher among men than women in all 36. As Fig. 1 shows, male and female obesity levels differed substantially in Albania, Bosnia and Herzegovina, Greece, Ireland, Israel, Latvia, Malta, and Serbia and Montenegro.

Evidence is increasing that the risk of cardiovascular and metabolic diseases associated with obesity is related to the amount and proportion of fat laid down in the abdomen, particularly at modest levels of excess body weight. Abdominal adiposity can be readily assessed by waist circumference measurements.

Children

Among primary school-age children (both sexes), the highest prevalence rates of overweight were in Portugal (7–9 years, 32%) Spain (2–9 years, 31%) and Italy (6–11 years, 27%); the lowest rates were in Germany (5–6 years, 13%), Cyprus (2–6 years, 14%) and Serbia and Montenegro (6–10 years, 15%) (Fig. 2).

For older children, few studies have measured weight and height and one must rely on reported data, mainly collected in two international studies. The Pro Children study, conducted in 2003 among 11-year-olds in nine European countries, showed a greater proportion of boys (17%) than girls (14%) being overweight *(8)*. The Health Behaviour in School-aged Children survey, conducted in 2001–2002 indicated that up to 24% of 13-year-old girls versus 34% of boys, and 31% of 15-year-old girls versus 28% of boys, were overweight (Fig. 3).

Up to 5% of both 13- and 15-year-old girls were obese, as were 9% of both 13- and 15-year-old boys *(9)*. A validation study conducted in Wales, United Kingdom in the context of the Health Behaviour in School-aged Children survey indicated that self-reported measures underestimate the true prevalence of overweight by about one quarter and of obesity by about one third in 13- and 15-year-olds *(10)*.

Trends over time

The prevalence of obesity has risen threefold or more since the 1980s, even in countries with traditionally low rates of overweight and obesity. Among both women and men, the prevalence of overweight in Ireland and the United Kingdom (England and Scotland) has risen rapidly, by more than 0.8 percentage points per year based

[1] Since this publication was written, the separation of Montenegro and Serbia has raised the number of countries in the Region to 53.

Fig. 1. Prevalence of overweight and obesity[a] among adults in countries in the WHO European Region based on surveys with an ending year of 1999 or later

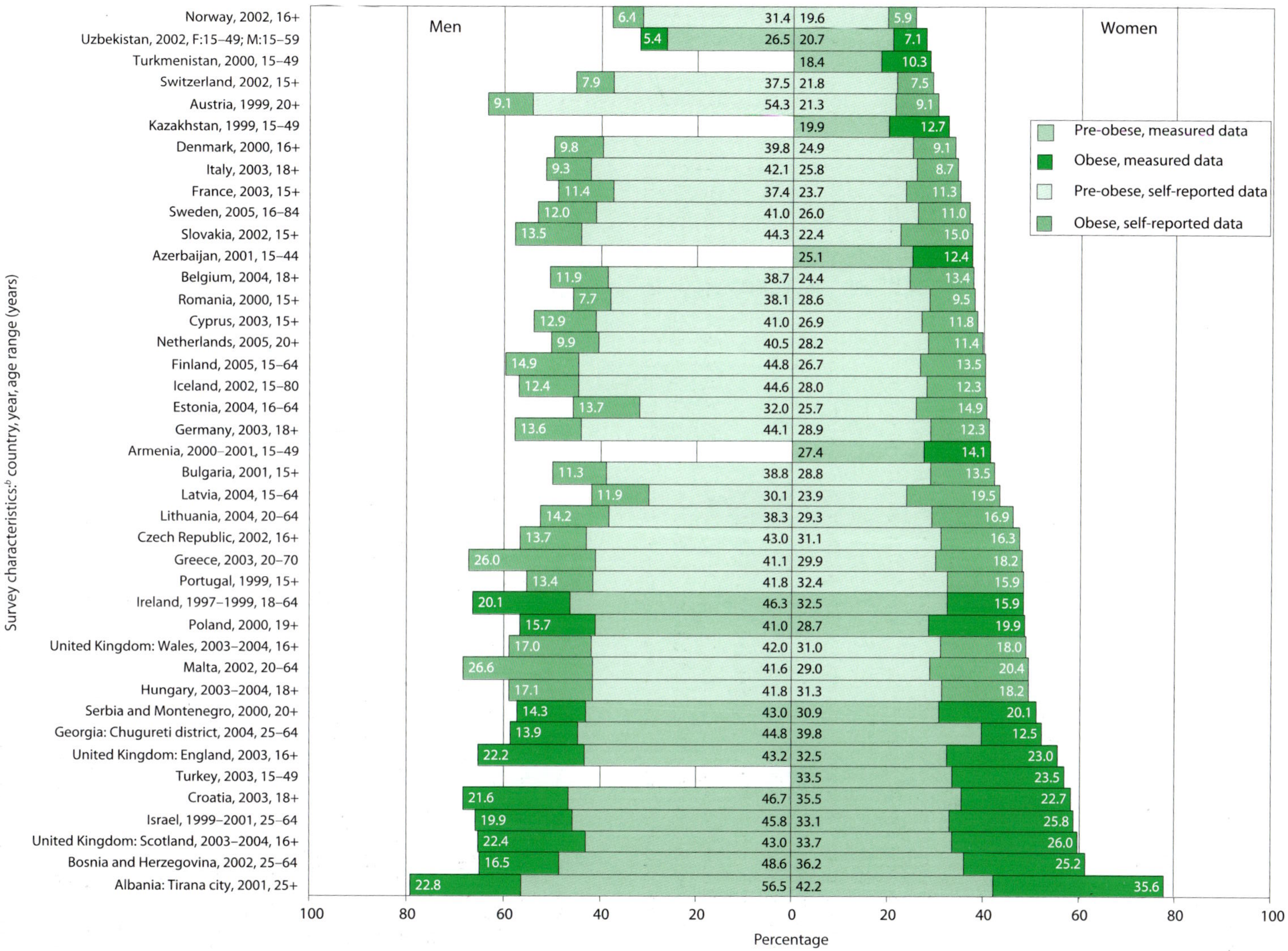

[a] Overweight is defined as BMI ≥ 25 kg/m² and obesity as BMI ≥ 30 kg/m² *(1)*. Overweight indicates pre-obese and obese.

[b] Intercountry comparisons should be interpreted with caution owing to different data collection methods, response rates, survey years and age ranges. The sources of data used can be provided on request.

Fig. 2. Prevalence of overweight and obesity[a] among children 11 years or younger in countries in the WHO European Region based on surveys with an ending year of 1999 or later

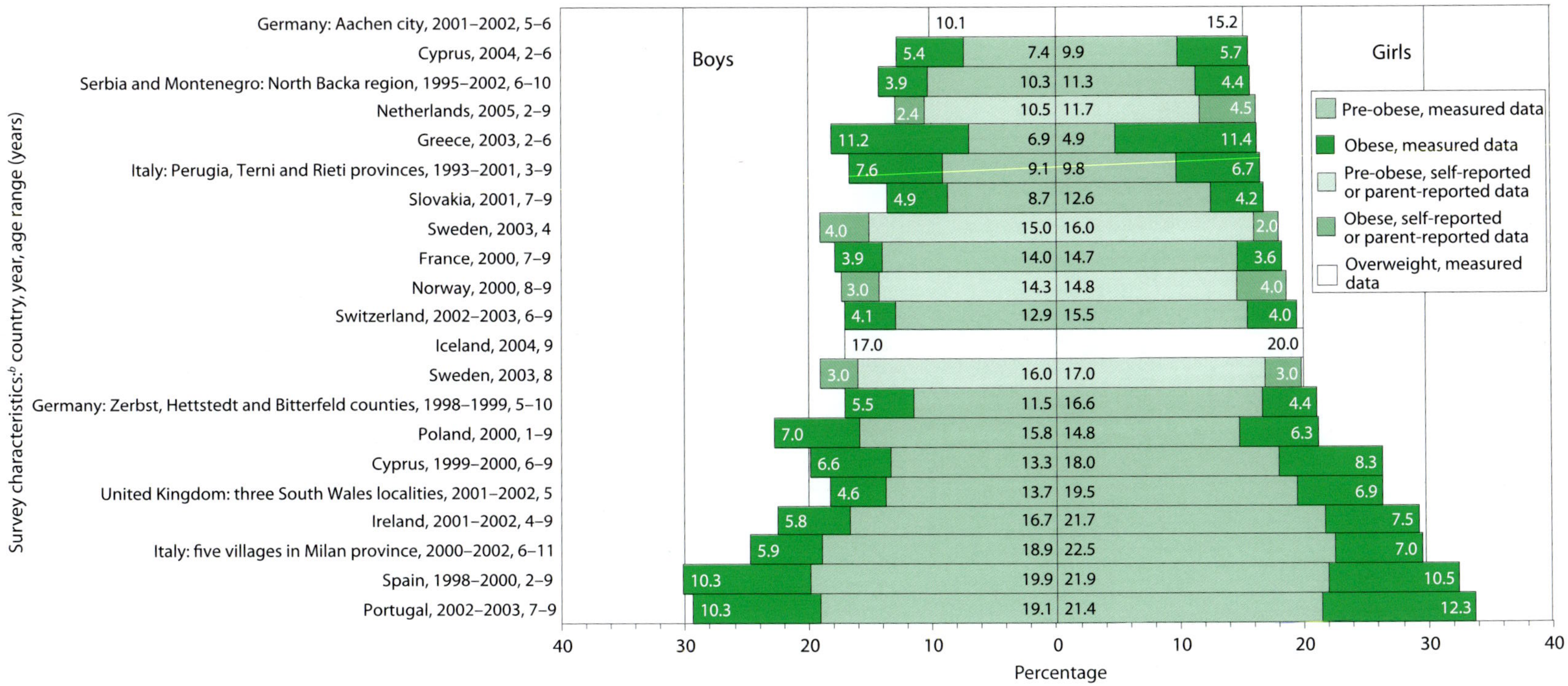

[a] Overweight and obesity are defined by using international age- and gender-specific cut-off points for BMI, passing through 25 kg/m² and 30 kg/m² by the age of 18 years, respectively *(3)*. Overweight includes pre-obese and obese.

[b] Intercountry comparisons should be interpreted with caution owing to different data collection methods, response rates, survey years and age ranges. The sources of data used can be provided on request.

Fig. 3. Prevalence of overweight[a] among 13-year-olds and 15-year-olds (based on self-reported data on height and weight) in countries in the WHO European Region, according to the 2001–2002 Health Behaviour in School-aged Children survey

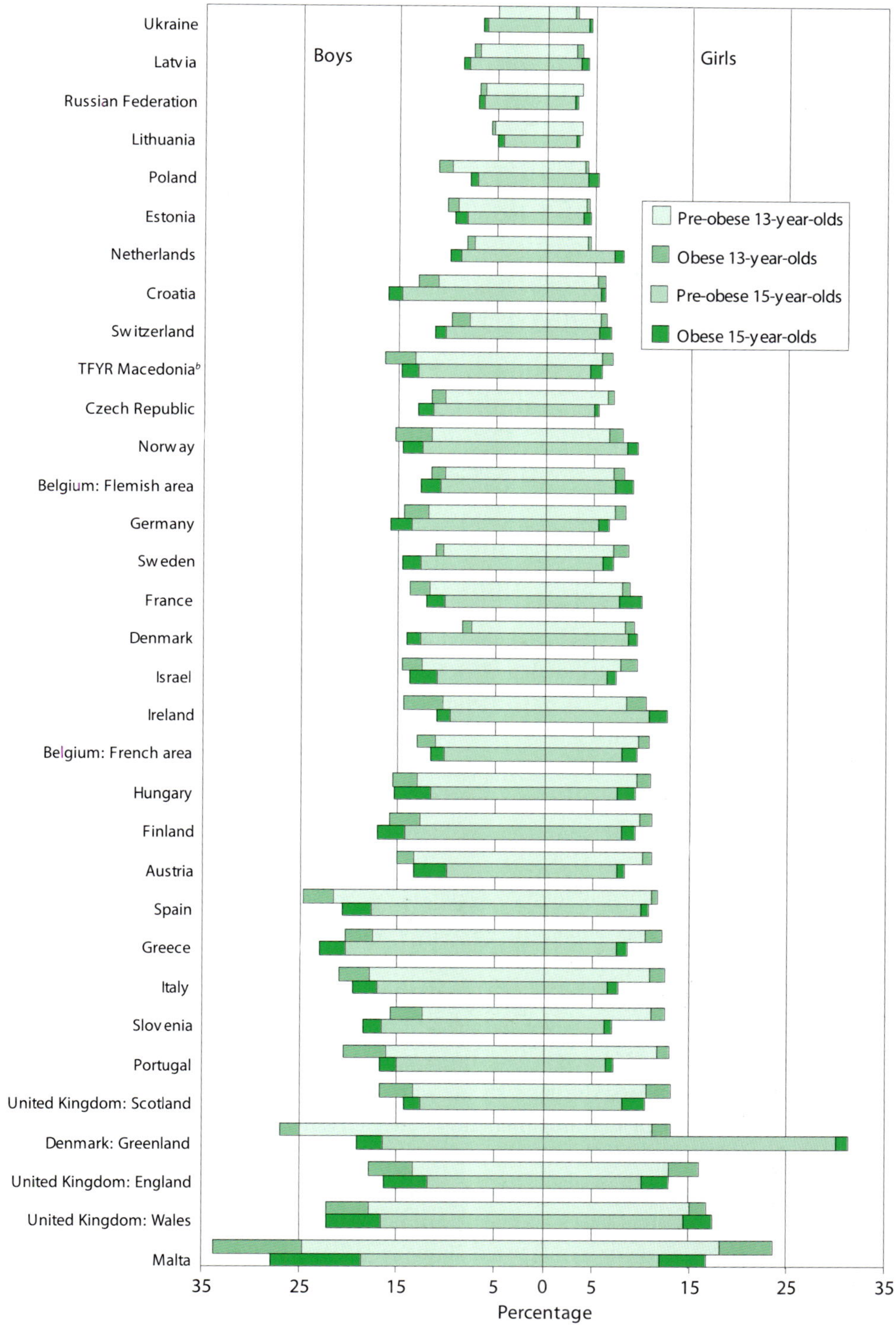

[a] Overweight and obesity defined by using international age- and gender-specific cut-off points for BMI, passing through 25 kg/m² and 30 kg/m² by the age of 18 years, respectively *(3)*. Overweight includes pre-obese and obese.

[b] The former Yugoslav Republic of Macedonia.

Source: Currie et al. *(9)*.

on measured data. Based on self-reported data, the highest annual increases in the prevalence of overweight in women and men were in Denmark (1.2 and 0.9 percentage points, respectively, from 1987 to 2001), Ireland (1.1 percentage points for both sexes from 1998 to 2002), France (0.8 percentage points among adults from 1997 to 2003), Switzerland (0.8 and 0.6 percentage points, respectively from 1992 to 2002) and Hungary (0.6 percentage points for both sexes from 2000 to 2004). In contrast, self-reported adult obesity rates have been falling in Estonia and Lithuania. If no action is taken and the prevalence of obesity continues to increase at the same rate as in the 1990s, an estimated 150 million adults will be overweight or obese by 2010 *(5)*.

The epidemic is progressing at especially alarming rates among children. In Switzerland, for example, overweight among children increased from 4% in 1960 to 18% in 2003. In England, United Kingdom the numbers increased from 8% to 20% between 1974 and 2003. In various regions of Spain, the prevalence of overweight more than doubled from 1985 to 2002 (Fig. 4). The only observed decrease in prevalence was in the Russian Federation during the economic crisis that followed the dissolution of the USSR. The annual increase in the prevalence of overweight in the countries with surveys portrayed in Fig. 5 averaged 0.1 percentage points during the 1970s, rising to 0.4 percentage points during the 1980s, 0.8 percentage points in the early 1990s and reaching as high as 2.0 percentage points in some countries by the 2000s. The International Obesity Task Force predicts that about 38% of school-age children in the WHO European Region will be overweight by 2010, and that more than a quarter of these children will be obese *(6)*.

Intergenerational influences

The mother's nutritional status before conception and her dietary intake during gestation have a major influence on fetal growth and development. Interactions between nutrients and genes during gestation restrict the range of body shapes in later life and influence the individual's ability to convert nutrients into lean and fat tissue.

This problem is likely to be very important in many countries in the WHO European Region where young women entering pregnancy have nutritional deficiencies, such as anaemia, inadequate essential fat stores and vitamin deficiencies; adolescent pregnancy is of particular concern as the competition for maternal and fetal growth may handicap the next generation.

In several countries in the Region, a sizeable proportion of the adult population were born under very disadvantageous conditions, with their mothers having meagre food sources during their pregnancies. There is increasing evidence of imprinting or programming of children's long-term responses to disease risks as a result of early fetal and childhood nutritional and other stresses. This may in part explain their greater susceptibility to type 2 diabetes and hypertension when as adults they put on modest amounts of weight. This emphasizes the importance of ensuring the well-being of adolescent girls and young women, as their health can affect the well-being of future generations.

Poor maternal nutrition is now recognized as a risk factor for the development of obesity, and particularly abdominal adiposity, among offspring. There are serious health risks for normal and, especially, underweight babies who subsequently experience rapid weight gain during early to middle childhood *(11)*. Thus, the conjunction of poor nutrition and undernutrition during early life with overweight, obesity and chronic noncommunicable disease in later life should be seen as a fundamentally connected aspect of ill health, and not as a question of first deficiency and then excess.

With the prevalence of obesity rising in the general population, the number of women who start pregnancy overweight and obese is also increasing. Obese mothers are much more likely to have obese children, especially if they have gestational diabetes or a pre-pregnancy metabolic syndrome, indicated by high serum insulin, high low-density lipoprotein (LDL) cholesterol, low high-density lipoprotein (HDL) cholesterol and high gestational weight gain. Increasing numbers of children are born with high birth weight (exceeding 4500 g or above the 95th percentile for standardized birth weight). A high birth weight is linked to later obesity, as shown in the cohorts born in Iceland in 1988 and 1994, in which the children who weighed above the 85th percentile at birth were more likely than others to be overweight at the ages of 6, 9 and 15 years *(12)*.

Fig. 4. Overweight among school-aged children in selected European countries based on surveys, 1958–2003

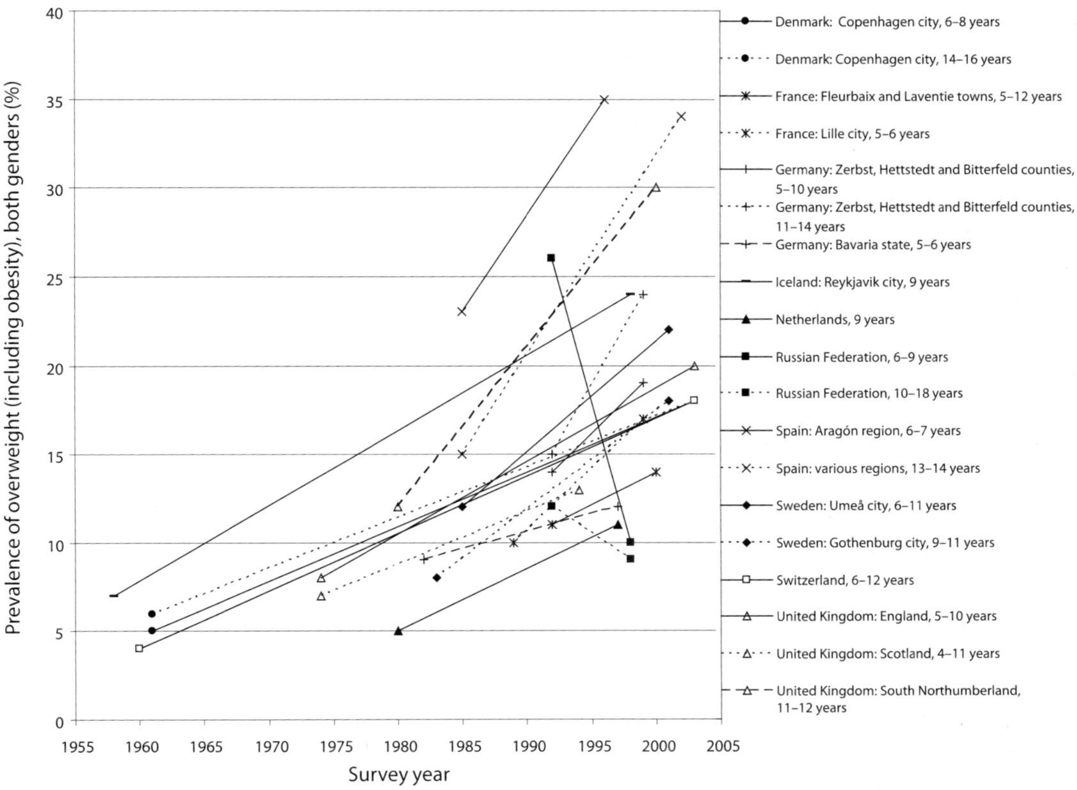

Fig. 5. Annual change in the prevalence of overweight among children and adolescents in selected European countries that conducted surveys, 1960–2005

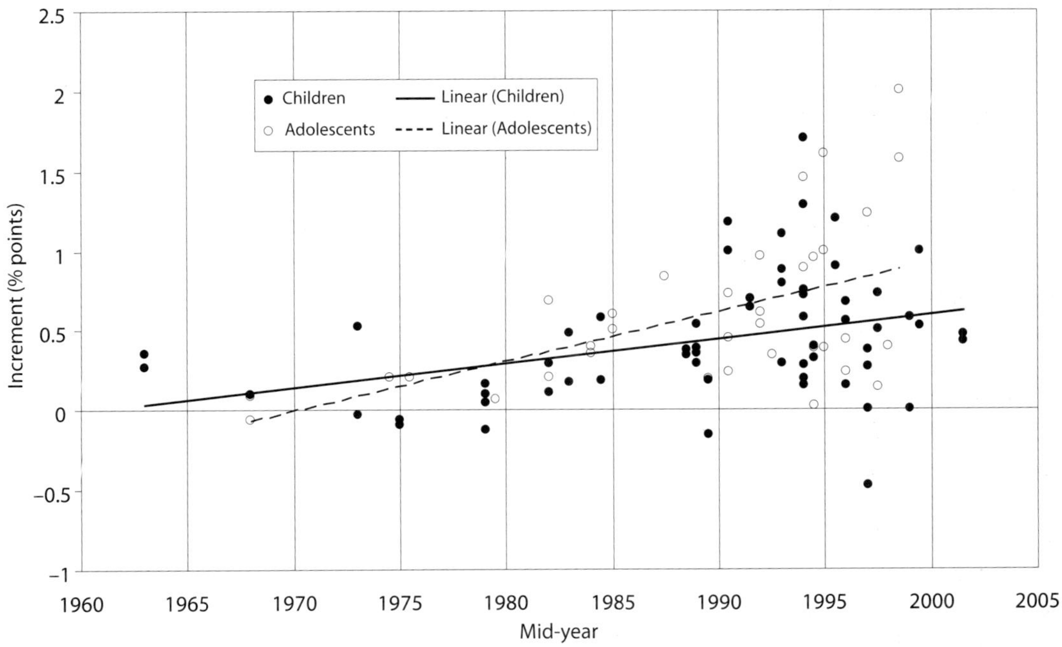

Sources: the sources of data used are available upon request.

Increasingly persuasive evidence now suggests that breastfeeding protects against obesity in the child. Lower levels of obesity are found among infants and young children breastfed from birth than formula-fed infants *(13)*. This evidence has therefore prompted the formulation of new growth standards, which should be based on the growth rate of exclusively breastfed children rather than formula fed children. New WHO Child Growth Standards *(4)* have been developed using this criterion and will highlight a previously unrecognized phenomenon of excess weight in early childhood.

If bigger babies have been bottle fed, become more overweight in childhood and then enter adolescence and adult life overweight or even obese, then many populations in Europe are set for an intergenerational amplification of the obesity and public health problem in ways not yet recognized by policy-makers. The increasing propensity for obesity to persist as children grow older (a feature known as tracking) implies that public health initiatives need to be taken at each stage of the life cycle. Fig. 6 models these effects into an intergenerational cycle that creates a vicious circle involving all age groups.

Fig. 6. The intergenerational cycle of overweight and obesity

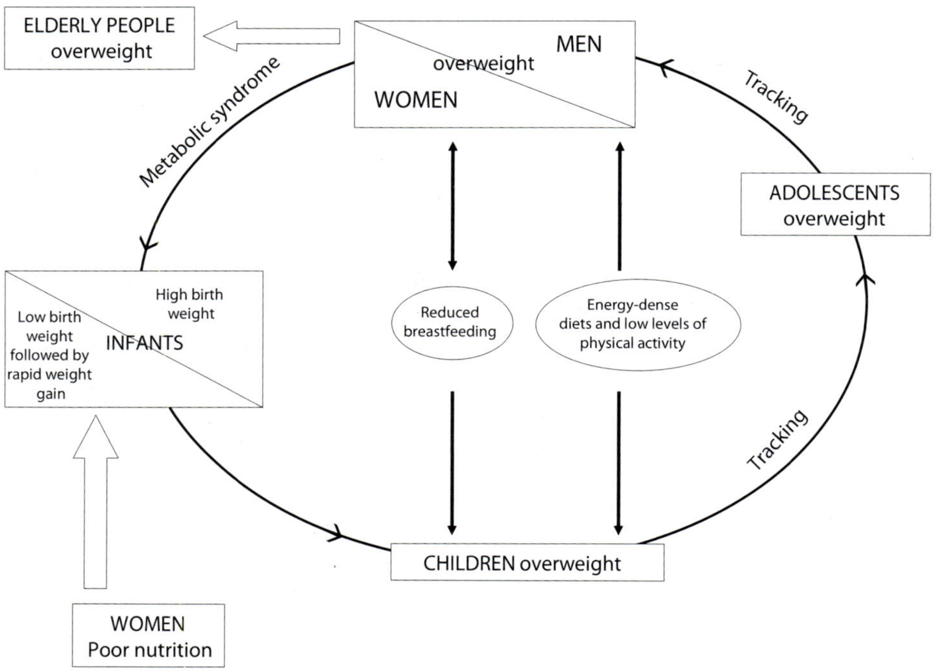

Public health effects

Obesity has considerable effects on morbidity and mortality. Type 2 diabetes and cardiovascular diseases, such as myocardial infarction and ischaemic stroke, are the two most important noncommunicable disease outcomes of obesity, as large epidemiological studies clearly describe. The term "metabolic syndrome" is increasingly used to describe the remarkable clustering of abdominal obesity with hypertension, dyslipidaemia and impaired insulin resistance; this problem affects 20–30% of the total population in the European Region. Other effects of obesity presented in recent literature include cancer at various sites, gallstones, narcolepsy, increased use of long-term medication, hirsutism, impaired reproductive performance, asthma, cataracts, benign prostatic hypertrophy, non-alcoholic steatohepatitis and musculoskeletal disorders such as osteoarthritis. Conversely, regular physical activity and normal weight are both important indicators of a decreased risk of mortality from all causes, cardiovascular diseases and cancer, with physical activity conferring a beneficial effect independent of BMI status.

An adult BMI above the optimum level (about 21–23 kg/m^2) is associated with a substantial burden of ill health, with the greatest disease-specific impact being the burden associated with the development of type 2 diabetes. Factors other than BMI contribute to disease risk, including tobacco smoking, alcohol consumption, excess salt intake, inadequate fruit and vegetable intake, and physical inactivity. Nevertheless, at least three quarters of type 2 diabetes, a third of ischaemic heart disease, a half of hypertensive disease, a third of ischaemic strokes and about a quarter of osteoarthritis can be attributed to excess weight gain. In addition, there is an impact on cancer development with nearly a fifth of colon cancers, a half of endometrial cancers and one in eight breast cancers in postmenopausal women being attributable to excess weight *(7)*.

The burden of disease attributable to excess BMI among adults in the European Region amounted to more than 1 million deaths and about 12 million life-years of ill health (disability-adjusted life-years – DALYs) in 2000 *(7)*. Gender differences have been described in the United States for the burden of disease attributable to obesity. Overweight and obese women suffer more illness than overweight and obese men, when compared to normal weight individuals, due to differences in physical, emotional and social well-being *(14)*.

With the obesity epidemic, the incidence of type 2 diabetes has been increasing and the condition is being diagnosed at progressively younger ages, as documented in the United States *(15)*.

Obesity reduces life expectancy. The Framingham study in the United States showed that obesity at age 40 years led to a reduction in life expectancy of 7 years in women and 6 years in men *(16)*. The United Kingdom Department of Health recently projected an average 5 years' lower life expectancy for men by 2050 if the current obesity trends continue *(17)* (Fig. 7). So far, no increase in cardiovascular disease mortality has been observed parallel to the increased prevalence of obesity, but this may be due to the increased use of drugs to counteract obesity risk factors or simply to the latency of the effect.

This analysis does not take account of the impact of childhood obesity. The health consequences of overweight for children during childhood are less clear, but a systematic review *(18)* shows that childhood obesity is strongly associated with risk factors for cardiovascular disease and diabetes, orthopaedic problems and mental disorders. A high BMI in adolescence predicts elevated adult mortality rates and cardiovascular disease, even if the excess

Fig. 7. Projected reductions in the average life expectancy at birth of males in the United Kingdom if obesity/overweight trends continue

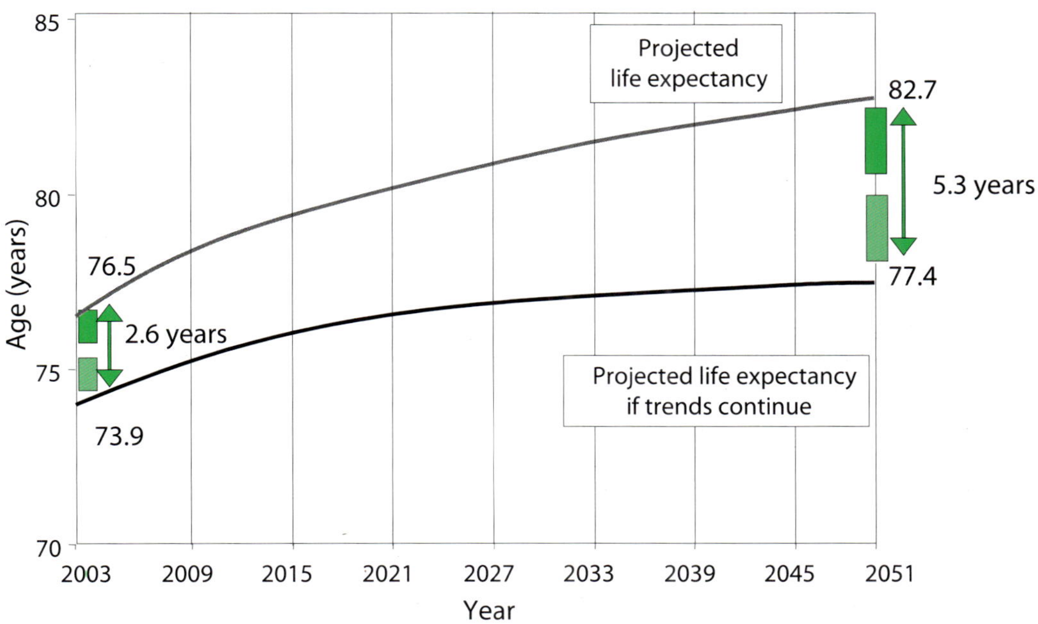

Source: Department of Health *(17)*.

body weight is lost. In most cases of adolescent overweight, however, the excess body weight is not lost. Many obesity-related health conditions once thought to be applicable only to adults are now being seen among children and with increasing frequency: examples include high blood pressure, early symptoms of hardening of the arteries, type 2 diabetes, non-alcoholic fatty liver disease, polycystic ovary disorder and disordered breathing during sleep *(18)*.

Obesity is also a feature of many adults with mental health conditions and/or with serious mental illness *(19)*, especially depressive and anxiety disorders *(20)*. Subgroups of obese people show abnormal patterns of food consumption, including uncontrolled binge eating, many of which would meet the criteria for binge eating disorder *(20)*. Personality disorder difficulties and pathology are more present in obese patients who binge eat than in those who do not *(21)*.

Economic consequences

Obesity imposes an economic burden on society through increased medical costs to treat the diseases associated with it (direct costs), lost productivity due to absenteeism and premature death (indirect costs) and missed opportunities, psychological problems and poorer quality of life (intangible costs). An estimate of the direct costs can be obtained through cost-of-illness studies, although the different methodologies used limit the possibility of cross-country comparisons.

A compilation of direct cost studies worldwide reveals that health expenditure per inhabitant attributable to obesity ranges between US$ 13 (United Kingdom, 1998) and US$ 285 (United States, 1998) (Table 1). Studies in the WHO European Region indicate that, in general, the direct health care costs of obesity account for 2–4% of national health expenditure *(1)*, but larger estimates have been made, owing to methodological differences. For instance, a study from Belgium *(22)* estimated the cost of obesity to be 6% of expenditure on social security, but the figure would be 3% if total current expenditure on health were the denominator.

Calculations in the United States indicate that people with a BMI exceeding 30 kg/m2 had 36% higher annual health care costs than those with BMI 20.0–24.9 kg/m^2, and that people with a BMI 25.0–29.9 kg/m^2 had 10% higher annual health care costs than those with BMI 20.0–24.9 kg/m^2 *(23)*. The cumulative costs of several major diseases measured over an eight-year period showed a close link with BMI: for men aged 45–54 years with a BMI of 22.5, 27.5, 32.5 or 37.5 kg/m^2, the cumulative costs were US$ 19 600, US$ 24 000, US$ 29 600 or US$ 36 500, respectively. Lifetime costs may of course be partly reduced by the premature death of obese people, but these costs may also be greater at older ages as the cumulative effects of prolonged obesity become apparent *(24)*.

The indirect costs include obese people's higher risk of being absent from work due to ill health or dying prematurely. Estimates of productivity losses in the United Kingdom (Table 1) indicate that these costs could amount to twice the direct health care costs. However, the economic and welfare losses due to obesity depend on the labour market situation and the structure of the social security system.

Recent estimates for Spain indicate that including the indirect costs due to the loss of productivity makes the total cost attributable to obesity an estimated €2.5 billion per year. This figure corresponds to 7% of the total health budget. The total direct and indirect annual costs of obesity in 2002 in the 15 countries that were European Union (EU) members before May 2004 were estimated to be €32.8 billion per year *(25)*. These estimates will be higher with the growing understanding of the health consequences of increased BMI in children and adults. The impact of pre-obese conditions in adults is also not usually considered. United Kingdom data indicate that, despite milder consequences, the widespread diffusion of pre-obesity would lead to a doubling of the estimated direct costs. Finally, none of the studies considers the cost of the consequences of overweight in children.

Expressed as a proportion of GDP, the total cost of obesity (direct and indirect) has been estimated to be 0.2% in Germany, 0.6% in Switzerland, 1.2% in the United States and 2.1% in China, thus suggesting that the effect is more pronounced in developing economies *(43)*.

Socioeconomic variation in prevalence

Several studies have noted an increased prevalence of overweight and obesity among specific population groups categorized by income level or educational attainment level (referred to generally as socioeconomic status)

Table 1. Estimated economic costs of obesity according to available studies

Country (study)	Year of estimate	BMI criterion	Cost			
			Type	Per capita (US$ at PPP[a])	Share of total current expenditure on health (%)	Share of GDP[b] (%)
In the WHO European Region						
Belgium *(22)*	1999	≥30	Direct	69	3	–
France (range) *(26)*	1992	≥30	Direct	71–148	0.6–1.3	–
France *(27)*	1992	≥27	Direct	202	1.8	0.9
Germany (range) *(28)*	2001	≥30	Direct	17–35	1.2–2.6	0.1–0.3
			Indirect	17–38	–	
Netherlands *(29,30)*	1993	≥30	Direct	32	1.7	–
Sweden *(31)*	2003	≥30	Direct	45	1.8	0.7
			Indirect	157	–	
Switzerland *(28)*	2001	≥25	Direct + indirect	186	–	0.6
United Kingdom (England, range) *(32)*	2002	≥30	Direct	NA[c]	2.3–2.6	–
EU (15 countries) *(25)*	2002	≥30	Direct + indirect	NA	NA	0.3
Outside the WHO European Region						
Australia (range) *(33)*	1995–1996	≥30	Direct	28–51	1.7–3.2	–
Canada *(34)*	1997	≥27	Direct	49	2.4	–
Canada *(35)*	2001	≥30	Direct	41	1.6	0.4
			Indirect	70	–	
Japan *(36)*	1995–1998	≥30	Direct	55	0.2	–
New Zealand *(37)*	1991	≥30	Direct	26	NA	–
United States *(38)*	1994	≥30	Direct	92	2.7	–
United States *(39)*	1995	≥30	Direct	263	7.3	–
United States *(40)*	1995	≥29	Direct	194	5.4	–
			Direct + indirect	371	–	1.4
United States *(41)*	1998	≥25	Direct	285	7.1	–
United States *(42)*	2000	≥30	Direct	199	4.8	1.2
			Indirect	183	–	

[a] PPP = purchasing power parity. PPP controls for differences in purchasing power, which means that a dollar may have more value in terms of consumption in one country than in another.

[b] When both direct and indirect costs have been calculated in the same study, the total cost as percentage of gross domestic product (GDP) is the sum of both direct and indirect costs.

[c] NA = not available.

(44,45). In most countries in the Region, obesity is more common among socially deprived communities, characterized by lower income, education and access to care. However, in some countries – such as Azerbaijan and Uzbekistan – obesity appears to be a greater burden for population groups with higher socioeconomic status.

Differences between countries indicate the role of economic development in the pattern of obesity. In low-income countries, obesity increases sharply as they grow richer, and the risk of obesity shifts from groups with higher socioeconomic status to those with lower. These trends may reflect the relative accessibility of mass-produced foods and drinks and decreasing manual labour as national income increases. In most countries, however, obesity is more prevalent among people of lower than high socioeconomic status, and the same appears to be true of type 2 diabetes. Other studies have suggested that social inequality may directly affect the health of disadvantaged people, and that this in turn, may be related to differential access to health promoting environments or to the psychosocial effects on health of perceived inequalities *(46,47)*.

Some evidence already points to the same problem of social disadvantage affecting the development of overweight in children *(48)*. In the United Kingdom, obesity among children aged 3 years has been reported to be more common among more deprived families in Scotland, and obesity among children aged 2–10 years tends to be more prevalent with increasing area deprivation and lower household income in England *(49)*. In addition, this problem has increased more rapidly over the last decade in more deprived families. Even the experience of low socioeconomic status during childhood strongly determines obesity in adulthood, regardless of whether the individual remains poor, so a coherent policy relating to social disadvantage needs to be incorporated into preventive strategies.

Gender, socioeconomic status and national characteristics may interact. In the Russian Federation, men with more education are more likely to be obese, whereas in the Czech Republic men with less education are more likely to be obese, yet in both countries women with less education are more likely to be obese *(50)*. The Health Survey for England, United Kingdom (1993–2001) found no clear BMI gradient by social class for men, but the prevalence of obesity was higher among women in a lower social class.

Obesity is also more common in some communities of recent immigration, although socioeconomic status may be responsible for some of these apparent differences. An investigation into the role of ethnicity in childhood obesity in Germany *(51)* found that known risk factors for overweight, especially poor education of the mother and watching more television, explained most of the difference in the prevalence of obesity by ethnic origin.

Finally, other risk factors, such as tobacco smoking and alcohol consumption, are also present to a larger extent in lower socioeconomic groups and thus a multiplicative effect is seen in the causation of noncommunicable diseases.

Assessing the challenge: the next steps

A robust monitoring system is needed to assess the physical measures of a nation's children and adults, not only to have a correct understanding of the progress of the epidemic but also to evaluate preventive initiatives that are progressively introduced. In Europe as a whole, the data available are currently inadequate for these purposes, and a system which assessed the relative effectiveness of different initiatives would be an invaluable service for all the Region's policy-makers.

More information will also be needed to highlight the burden of ill health due to pre-obese conditions and to children's overweight. Lastly, a better understanding of the implications of the obesity epidemic on health budgets and on overall economic development will provide a more comprehensive basis for decision-making.

2. The determinants of obesity

Main messages

- The simultaneous presence of physical inactivity and poor diet to a large extent explains the obesity epidemic. About two thirds of adults in the western part of the European Region are not physically active at recommended levels, and people's diets are characterized by high energy density and low satiating power.
- Dietary practices differ between countries in the Region, but time trends show that these differences are narrowing. Mediterranean countries have been characterized by high consumption of plant foods, vegetable oils and fish, but this traditional pattern has been disappearing, especially among younger people.
- Exclusive breastfeeding and appropriate complementary feeding practices protect against the development of obesity. Large sectors of the population still do not follow such optimal infant feeding practices.
- A wide range of environmental factors influences individual energy intake and expenditure, including family practices, school policies and procedures, transport and urban planning policies, commercial marketing activities and policies on food supply and agriculture. People experience many aspects of the environment as being obesogenic: encouraging dietary or physical activity behaviour that increases the risk of obesity.
- Families and schools, including kindergartens, have a special role to play in establishing high-quality eating and physical activity habits, as well as in teaching children about healthy behaviour. They should provide environments supportive of healthy eating and activity patterns. This is not the case, however, in most countries in the European Region.
- Children are vulnerable to commercial food marketing; this includes a wide range of methods, in addition to television advertising, which can bypass parental control.
- Joining the labour force is a time of lifestyle change that may lead to weight gain. Most labour is now sedentary and, if good catering facilities and adequate time for meals are not available, people may have recourse to energy-dense quick snacks.
- Food manufacturers and suppliers, including fast-food outlets, are driving food consumption through the design, portion size and pricing of food products.
- Agricultural policy influences dietary patterns through the relative pricing and availability of different types of food. For decades, policies were geared to producing ever cheaper fats, sugars and animal products; countering these longstanding effects is a major policy challenge.
- Consumers want informative nutrition labelling, but find current labelling systems confusing and sometimes misleading. Labelling that provides an appropriate illustration of good nutritional profiles of foods could be a major incentive for the consumption of healthier products.
- Specific social groups are especially vulnerable to obesogenic environments. People with lower socioeconomic status face structural, social, organizational, financial and other constraints in making healthy lifestyle choices. In particular, food prices and availability significantly influence dietary choices.

Introduction

The imbalance between energy intake and expenditure is the outcome of contemporary social trends. At least two thirds of the adults in the EU countries are insufficiently physically active for optimal health *(52)*. A large proportion of the population also consumes too many energy-dense, nutrient-poor foods and drinks *(53)* and not enough fruit and vegetables *(54)*.

Understanding why people might consume excess energy and might not expend enough energy to prevent weight gain requires examining the upstream influences on dietary intake and physical activity behaviour.

Upstream influences can be considered in terms of a series of causes; some of these are immediately reflected in behaviour patterns, while others are more distant and shape the context rather than behaviour itself. Fig. 8 illustrates an ecological model describing the influences on energy expenditure and food intake. The vertical and horizontal links may vary in different societies and populations.

Fig. 8. Societal policies and processes directly and indirectly influencing the prevalence of obesity

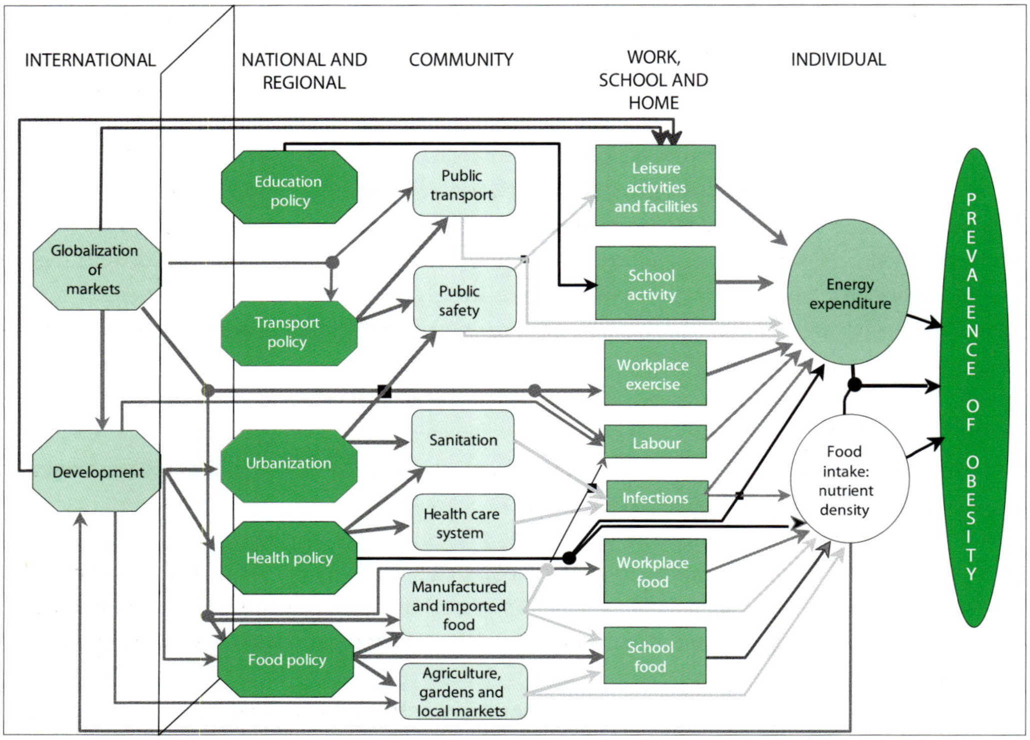

Source: adapted from Kumanyika et al. *(55)*.

This chapter considers specific aspects of this general model: the determinants of food choices and physical activity behaviour in different settings, across different social groups and at different points in the life cycle. The discussion shows that the determinants of obesity and of an obesogenic (obesity-causing) environment lie across a broad range of sectors and result from policies in agriculture, trade, education and planning, as much as in health and social welfare.

Sedentary behaviour, physical activity, fitness and obesity

Body fat accumulates when the energy content of the food and drinks consumed exceeds the energy expended by an individual's metabolism and physical activity. Since both intake and output contribute to weight gain, it is often difficult to identify either excess intake or physical inactivity as the sole and clearly demonstrable factor responsible for an individual's or a society's obesity problem *(56)*. Further, as weight gain begins to impose higher cardiovascular and respiratory demands, as well as backache, arthritis and sweating when exercising, weight gain itself may lead to less activity. Claiming that poor diet or sedentary behaviour is selectively responsible for a country's health burden is therefore inappropriate; both need to be improved.

Physical activity is of benefit at all weights because it:

- reduces the likelihood of cardiovascular diseases, hypertension and type 2 diabetes;
- beneficially influences fat and carbohydrate metabolism, enhancing insulin sensitivity and improving blood lipids; and
- can increase muscle mass, even when the change in weight is small or nonexistent *(57)*.

Physical activity is better at improving weight stability than weight loss, so, once people have lost weight by changing their diets they need to have developed a consistent habit of greater daily activity. Even moderate physical activity can substantially reduce the risk of diabetes *(58)* and most other major chronic diseases.

There is a consensus on the amount of physical activity needed for beneficial effects. Moderately intensive activity, such as fast walking for 30 minutes five days per week, clearly reduces the likelihood of developing both cardiovascular disease and type 2 diabetes among adults. Longer periods of activity, such as 60–90 minutes of walking or activities at higher intensities per day, are now proposed to combat weight gain in countries with obesogenic diets.

At least two thirds of the adults in the EU countries appear not to reach recommended levels of physical activity *(52)*. The activity level has decreased in recent decades, mainly because environments have discouraged it more and more. These environments include transport, housing, workplaces and schools, as well as leisure-time settings.

Thus, even if physical activity alone is not very effective in reducing weight, strong evidence supports urgent action to increase physical activity across the whole European Region.

Determinants of physical activity

Several aspects of the social environment (such as school policies or the media) and the built environment (such as transport and urban design) influence physical activity choices.

1. Schools in many countries are placing more emphasis on academic tasks, often at the expense of time for physical education and other forms of physical activity. In addition, in free time during the day, activities involving exercise are increasingly competing with sedentary activities such as television watching (in younger classes) or computer use.
2. Fewer children cycle and walk to school in many countries, mostly because of parents' safety concerns.
3. The availability of multiple television channels throughout the day and the high popularity of electronic entertainment make the sedentary use of leisure time almost a default at most ages.
4. For adults, the use of private cars has increased in recent decades, while physically active means of transport (such as cycling and walking) are at historically low levels in many countries.
5. Participation in some traditional sports has decreased recently, in part owing to demographic changes and the increase in the variety of sports disciplines. Commercial fitness clubs and activities have developed, but their accessibility may be limited in some areas and for some population groups.
6. Physical activity during work has decreased, with increasing numbers of employees in sedentary occupations. The sociocultural environment provided by employers is an important determinant of the physical activity behaviour of employees. This includes, for instance, offering opportunities for physical activity in the occupational setting itself and incentives to promote participation in sports and fitness activities or active commuting.
7. Urban design and the urban physical environment can facilitate or constrain physical activity and active living. Design that reduces the spatial separation of living, working, shopping and leisure activities reduces travel distances, acting as an incentive for cycling and walking. Several European cities have good examples of urban design to encourage cycling and incentives to promote the use of bicycles instead of, or in addition to, other forms of transport.

8. In residential neighbourhoods, not only the physical availability of possibilities for exercise but also the maintenance level, aesthetic quality and perceived safety and security of public spaces can affect people's willingness to be physically active. Socioeconomic status is an important factor in these relationships, both through the accessibility of the facilities (as a result of equipment cost, entry cost and location) or people's perceived competence to use them.

Although most changes in recent decades have not supported more physical activity, each of these settings provides great potential to promote it. Modifiable determinants of sustainable transport solutions include road safety, a more equitable distribution of investment in the transport sector, and price "signals" favouring non-motorized and public transport.

At the individual level, further determinants shape the use of physical activity resources. Studies of the reluctance of schoolchildren to participate in sports, for example, show that many, especially those who are already overweight, dislike both competitive sports or activities where they are likely to fail and the need to change clothing in communal spaces or to wear clothing (such as swimming outfits) that exposes them to peer ridicule. Some cultures have belief systems that explicitly restrict body exposure in public, especially for women and girls, and alternative opportunities for activity need to be considered.

Dietary influences on obesity

The modern food environment provides a wide range of opportunities to consume food and drink products. These are then readily consumed, which inadvertently leads to what has been described as "passive overconsumption", where the individual has no way of recognizing that he or she is consuming particularly energy-dense products. The recent analyses of different studies on individual responses to food, assessing spontaneous intake in both carefully controlled environments *(59,60)* and everyday life, all point to two dietary factors that are particularly conducive to inadvertent overeating:

- the consumption of very energy-dense diets: high in energy per unit weight because extra fat and/or sugars have been added, because the food has been refined to limit its water-holding and bulking properties or because fruit and vegetables are marginally present; and
- the consumption of energy-rich drinks, such as sugary drinks, between meals.

These two factors seem to evade the normal biological short-term regulation of appetite and food intake, so children and adults tend not to adjust their intakes when these foods and drinks are constantly offered. This problem is then accentuated in sedentary societies, where people need to eat less in general and where maintaining an energy balance when energy-dense foods and drinks are consumed is therefore more difficult.

Conversely, diets low in energy density, with lower proportions of fat, more complex carbohydrates and more fibre, protect against weight gain *(61)*. Intervention studies also show that a high intake of dietary fibre may assist in losing weight *(62)*. Such low-energy diets, however, should have an adequate density of micronutrients and bioactive compounds to supply the required micronutrients while keeping the energy intake low.

Given this perspective, the emergence of sweetened beverages *(63)* and "fast food"[2] *(64)* as specific risk factors is not surprising. In addition, large portion sizes of energy-dense foods increase the risk of excessive consumption *(65)*, while the frequency of eating itself has not been shown to contribute specifically to weight change, when the type of food is the same. Thus, the findings that higher fruit and vegetable intakes are linked to lower weight gains *(66)* and that a high meat (with its associated fat) intake is linked to a greater risk of weight gain *(67)* are not surprising. There is some evidence that alcohol contributes to obesity in men, but no consistent association. Some recent evidence links weight gain to foods with a high glycaemic index, but longer-term studies are needed to confirm this.

[2] Defined here as food such as hamburgers, pizza and fried chicken eaten outside the home in self-service outlets.

Although many cited reports seem to contradict these conclusions, care needs to be taken with their interpretation, because many studies rely on self-reported intakes and even weight gains, and both measures are subject to large errors. This leads to marked underreporting of total energy, fat and sugar intakes, especially in those most overweight *(68)*.

Dietary habits in Europe and their relation to obesity

Dietary patterns in the WHO European Region may be discerned by means of data on food supplies, food sales, household purchases and individual consumption (usually using self-reported diaries). The results are summarized below.

1. The proportion of total fat in the diet of adults ranges from about 30% to more than 40% of energy intake (15–30% of total energy from fat is currently recommended). This is high in almost all European countries, especially in Greece and Belgium (adults) (Fig. 9) and in Spain and France (children). Vegetable oil is widely available in southern European countries, whereas both vegetable oil and animal fat are widely available in western and northern Europe. The intake of simple carbohydrates is also greater than the currently recommended 10% of total energy in most countries.
2. Fruit and vegetable supply has increased during the past four decades in the European Region. Southern Europe has the highest consumption levels, although consumption has declined in some countries during the past decade, while several northern European countries have recorded an increase. In many countries, mean individual consumption levels remain substantially below the recommended minimum of 400 g per day (Fig. 9).
   - Low fruit and vegetable intake and inadequate amounts of whole-grain cereals account for the surprisingly uniformly low intake of dietary fibre in European countries: 1.8–2.4 g/MJ for men and 2.0–2.8 g/MJ for women. Recommended intakes are 2.5–3.1 g/MJ.
   - Mediterranean countries have had higher consumption of plant foods, vegetable oil and fish, but the traditional pattern has been disappearing, especially among young people. Data on dietary trends (Fig. 10) show that southern European countries are losing their advantageous diets and becoming more like northern and western Europe in their inappropriate diets.
3. Countries differ greatly in the consumption of sugar-rich beverages (soft drinks). Consumption is lower in southern Europe than in northern Europe, and men consume more than women. In all countries except Germany and Greece, availability has increased over the past decade (Fig. 10).
4. The European Region has the highest alcohol consumption in the world, particularly among men *(69)*. Wine is generally preferred in southern Europe, while beer is consumed more in central and northern Europe. In the past four decades, the supply of beer has increased within the EU, whereas that of wine has decreased.

These data indicate that both factors conducive to the risk of excess energy intake are in general present in the European Region:

- a diet characterized by high energy density and low satiating power (feeling of fullness after eating) due to a high proportion of energy from fat, a high intake of sugar and a low intake of fibre; and
- rising consumption of sugar-rich beverages, in parallel with sustained consumption of alcoholic beverages.

The food environment

The context in which people eat influences the nature and amount of food eaten. Home and school environments have been most extensively studied, although other settings have also been examined.

Fig. 9. Proportion of energy from fat and from fruits and vegetables among men and women in selected European countries from individual-based surveys, 1992–2004

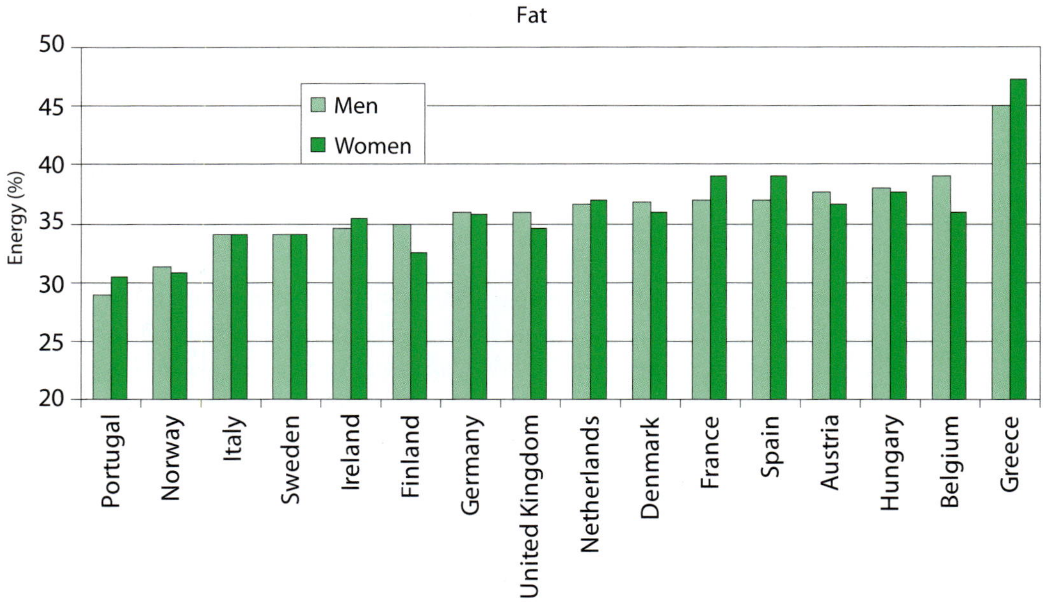

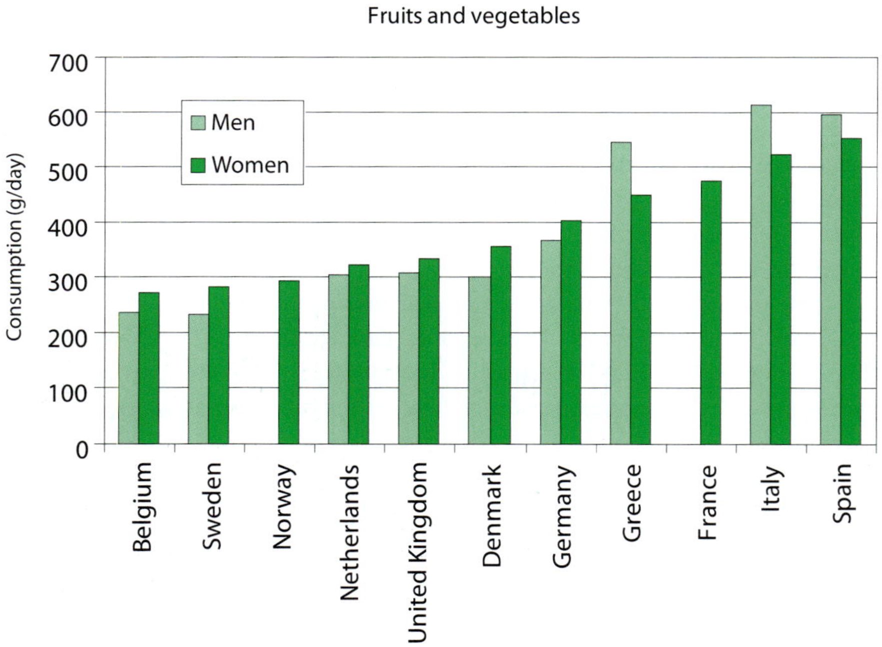

Note. The surveys of fruit and vegetable consumption in France and Norway were among women only.

Sources: Elmadfa & Weichselbaum *(53)*, Harrington et al. *(70)*, Netherlands Nutrition Centre *(71)*, Agudo et al. *(54)*, de Vriese et al. *(72)*.

Homes

There is strong evidence that having overweight or obese parents raises the risk of obesity, independent of genetic factors. In addition, evidence shows an increased risk of obesity developing among children in families where the parents show poor control of dietary intake, there are fewer or infrequent family meals, television is

Fig. 10. Trends in the mean household availability of soft drinks and fruits and vegetables per person per day in selected European countries

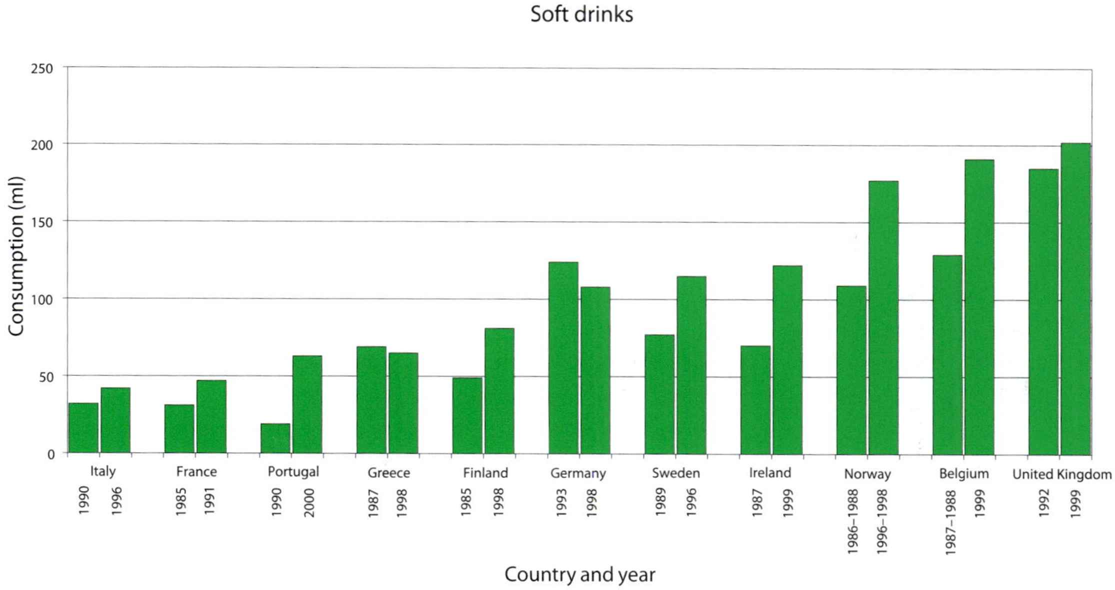

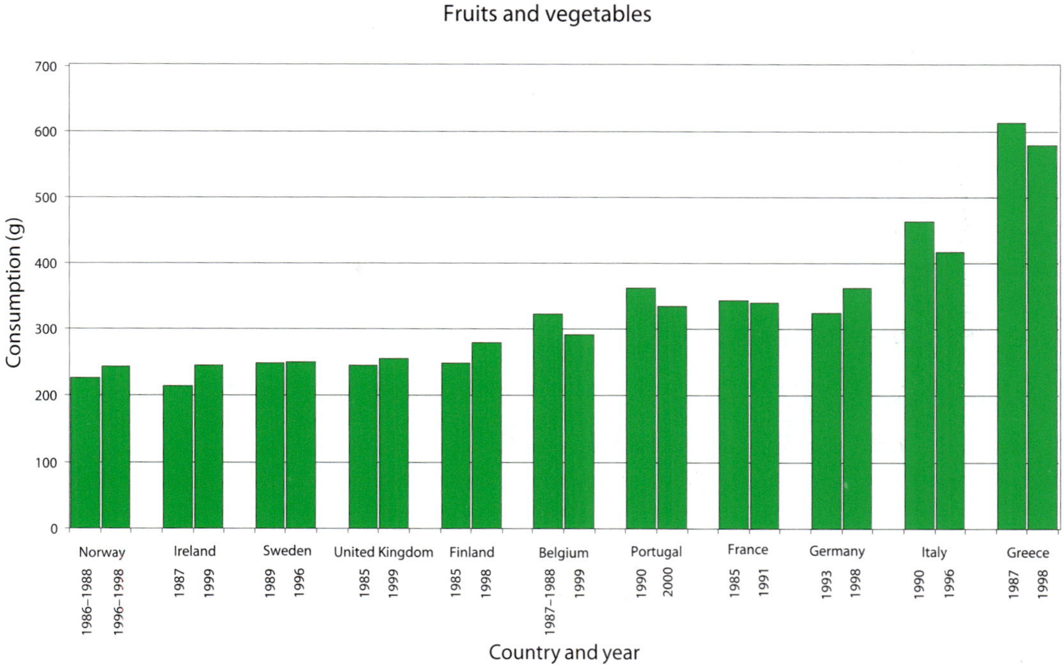

Source: DAFNE Data Food Networking *(73)*.

watched during meals, there is frequent snacking or the mother undergoes episodic weight-loss dieting. Obesity among children is also linked to a lower socioeconomic status of the family and having a single parent. Despite the frequent opportunities to consume food outside the home, the importance of the home environment should not be overlooked.

Schools

The school food environment includes the meals provided, vending machines and other sources of food in the school, policies relating to the food brought into school and the availability of drinking-water free of charge. Moderate evidence demonstrates that the school food environment influences dietary intake and potentially promotes unhealthy eating habits that favour the development of obesity among students. Good evidence also indicates that programmes adopting a whole-school approach of integrating policies on food with those on education and physical activity, and of involving parents and students in developing policy, can improve dietary patterns. Interventions providing information and offering price incentives have been shown to influence dietary choices (with price incentives being especially effective), but the changes were not sustained when the incentives were withdrawn *(74)*.

Workplaces

Entering the workforce is associated with lifestyle change that may induce an increase in body weight. There is limited evidence on which workplace factors are related to dietary habits that favour the development of obesity; these may include a decrease in routine daily physical activity and the selection of foods available at workplace canteens/cafeterias. On the other hand, workplaces may provide opportunities for preventive programmes aimed at adopting healthy behaviours. Educational activities combined with improved catering and physical activity promotion programmes have great potential.

Food retailers

Marketing incentives strongly influence food purchasing behaviour (see the discussion on marketing and advertising on pp. 21–22). For lower-income households especially, food choices may be influenced by pricing strategies and by the accessibility of local shops and supermarkets, and accessibility in turn is influenced by the location of retailers and the transport services available in both urban and rural areas. In some countries, the expression "food deserts" has been introduced to describe areas of poor accessibility.

Food service outlets

Eating meals outside the home is increasingly popular in many societies. Moderate evidence links frequent eating in restaurants and/or fast-food outlets to higher intakes of energy and fat among adults and adolescents. Further, limited evidence shows that the presence of fast-food outlets and restaurants is associated with an elevated prevalence of obesity in local areas.

What drives the food environment

Observations on the home, school, workplace and other local settings should be viewed in context. Specifically, many factors shape the food market, including agriculture and trade policy, and the prevailing availability, price and labelling of food. Interventions in production, distribution and pricing in Finland and Norway have been shown to influence consumption patterns and lead to improvements in population health.

Food availability

The rising availability of energy-dense foods is believed to be a prime driver of the obesity epidemic. As incomes rise and populations become more urban, societies enter into "nutrition transition", characterized by a shift from diets featuring grains and vegetables to those high in fat and sugar, an increasing number of meals eaten outside the home and a greater proportion of processed foods.

Changes in food production systems, transport, processing and packaging, and larger portion sizing facilitate the consumption of energy-dense foods, but they can also increase the availability of fruits and vegetables. Food can be bought in many places and around the clock, and the most accessible products have the highest energy density.

Multinational producers and retailers mediate the nutrition transition by entering new markets and by developing global brand names and marketing strategies, resulting in producer-induced demand.

Agriculture and trade policy

Agricultural policies such as the EU Common Agricultural Policy have encouraged the production of sugar, fats and oils, meat and alcohol at low cost through subsidies and other measures, and limited the market supply of fruit and vegetables.

Food surpluses (of butter, for example) have induced marketing measures to increase consumption, and this has led to excessive domestic consumption and distortion of international trade, with negative health effects in both high- and low-income countries.

Nutrition goals and recommendations adopted at the pan-European level – especially about sugar, fat, alcohol, and fruit and vegetables – could be used to guide policy measures concerning agricultural production, trade, processing, retailing (including catering) and marketing.

Food prices

The real price of food is the lowest in history for many countries in the European Region. Food accounts for a declining share of household budgets in most countries in the Region. However, people with low incomes are more price sensitive than those with higher incomes and therefore react more strongly to price changes.

Food labelling

Consumers find current nutrition label formats generally confusing but respond well to brief health claims and nutrition symbols on food. Preliminary experience in the United Kingdom has indicated that highlighting the macronutrient composition of processed foods with a signposting system may better guide consumers' choice. Health claims may also direct consumers' choice more easily.

Consumer organizations want nutrition labelling to be mandatory and EU-wide; the nutrients labelled should be those that are most important for public health. Mandatory labelling gives the food industry an incentive to develop healthier products.

Food marketing and advertising

As discussed above, dietary choices depend on a range of external factors, including price, availability and adequate information about products, as well as individuals' personal preferences and cultural values. The promotional activities of food and beverage companies can utilize all these factors: prices (such as special offers and discounts), availability (such as numerous retail outlets with energy-dense and nutrient-poor food conveniently located at the checkout), information (generally through food advertising and specifically through, for example, health claims and nutritional labelling), personal taste (such as using colouring or flavouring additives in the foods) and cultural values (such as using celebrities and sports personalities in product promotions).

WHO *(75)* considered the evidence on the nature and strength of the links between diet and noncommunicable diseases and classified as "probable" or "convincing" the adverse effect of heavy marketing of energy-dense foods and fast-food outlets. A recent WHO forum and technical meeting *(76)* reviewed the area of marketing food and non-alcoholic beverages to children and concluded that the commercial promotion of energy-dense micronutrient-poor foods and beverages can adversely affect children's nutritional status.

Intensive marketing of energy-dense, nutrient-poor foods can undermine healthy lifestyle choices. Current policies focus on marketing directed to children, but they should also consider adults, as their competence to make healthy choices or their capacity to resist the marketing of unhealthy food may not fully protect them from the damage to health that such marketing may inflict.

Several surveys have noted that the great majority of food advertisements, especially those shown during children's television programmes, encourages the consumption of energy-dense foods and beverages. A systematic review of the scientific evidence, conducted for the United Kingdom Food Standards Agency in 2003 *(77)*, concluded that sufficient evidence shows that advertising increases the overall consumption of food categories, as well as choices between brands. A review by the United States Institute of Medicine in 2006 *(78)* found strong evidence that advertising has short-term effects on the overall diet of children aged 2–11 years and moderate evidence of long-term effects on children aged 6–11 years. This review also noted strong statistical evidence linking higher exposure to television advertising and obesity among children aged 2–11 years and adolescents aged 12–18 years. Children's exposure to television advertising of energy-dense foods is associated with an elevated prevalence of overweight, and exposure to the advertising of healthier foods is weakly linked to a reduced prevalence of overweight *(79)*.

New forms of advertising are increasingly being used that bypass parental control and target children directly. These include Internet promotion (using interactive games, free downloads, blogs and chatterbots), SMS (short message service) texting to children's mobile phones, product promotions in schools and preschools, and brand advertising in educational materials. New forms of advertising are invading public areas, such as on-screen advertising in public transport and interactive electronic hoardings (billboards).

In the past decade, the marketing of foods and beverages has grown rapidly in the eastern part of the European Region, linked to high levels of foreign direct investment in that area's food and beverage sector, especially in confectionery, soft drinks and snack foods.

Socioeconomic drivers of obesity

The section on socioeconomic variations in overweight and obesity (pp. 10–12) noted increased prevalence among population groups with lower income or educational attainment. People of low socioeconomic status live in environments where the described determinants of obesity are present to a larger extent, and they are less equipped to counteract obesogenic influences.

Lower socioeconomic status seems to be correlated with the markers of poor diet associated with obesity, such as lower consumption of fresh fruit and vegetables, reduced breastfeeding rates and higher intake of energy-dense foods. Surveys conducted in high-income countries show that adults and children with lower socioeconomic status tend to be more sedentary than those with higher status, potentially owing to the lower availability and affordability of facilities and activities, less leisure time, and poorer knowledge and fewer positive attitudes about the benefits of exercise *(80)*.

In less economically developed countries, much of the population may have a high degree of food insecurity, such that a large proportion of household income is spent acquiring food, and people may be experiencing a nutrition transition. Traditional labour-intensive occupations and domestic activities can be replaced by more sedentary behaviour. Urbanization is likely to increase exposure to and marketing of energy-dense and nutrient-poor food products, decrease walking and increase sedentary leisure activities.

Surveillance systems for monitoring the determinants of obesity need to be developed that are sensitive to effects on vulnerable groups, such as people experiencing socioeconomic deprivation and those in the very early stages of life.

Steps should also be taken to identify simple, comparable measures of diet and physical activity, given the evidence that the majority of Europe's population needs to change both these contributors to the obesity epidemic.

Comparisons across countries suggest that, at least in the 50 countries with the highest level of development, the prevalence of obesity (and of type 2 diabetes) is linked to the degree of inequality in society (measured using such indicators as the Gini coefficient), rather than the absolute level of income or educational attainment *(81)*. This suggests that the prevailing social climate can affect individuals' perceived opportunity to improve their health, or perceived control over their ability to do so, and may increase their sense of fatalism about their health.

Lower socioeconomic status not only increases the risk of obesity but may result from obesity. Several studies have noted that obesity increases time off school and reduces the numbers of social relationships among adolescents, perceived popularity among child and adolescent peers, school educational attainment and employment prospects, resulting in a greater likelihood of an occupation with lower income or unemployment *(82)*. Thus, social isolation, lower education and lower income may exacerbate the relationship between lower socioeconomic status and obesity.

Obesity and mental health

Social determinants of obesity such as poverty and area deprivation are also associated with mental disorders such as depression and schizophrenia. Mental health problems are also risk factors for obesity in their own right, and there are strong associations between some of these disorders – such as depression *(83)* and schizophrenia *(84,85)* – and obesity *(86)*. A contributing factor is that some of the medication prescribed for mental health problems can cause weight gain *(87,88)*.

In addition, strong evidence relates poor self-esteem to obesity *(89)*, especially in children and adolescents *(90)*. Obese girls are more likely to suffer from serious emotional problems and hopelessness *(91)*.

Clinical and community studies have described an association between depression and obesity. Children and adolescents with major depressive disorder may be at increased risk of developing overweight, and obese people seeking weight-loss treatment may have elevated rates of mood disorders. Obesity is associated with major depressive disorder in females; however, most overweight and obese people in the community do not have mood disorders *(92)*.

Studying the determinants: the next steps

Steps should be taken to provide comparable data on dietary consumption and on physical activity levels, given the evidence that the majority of Europe's population needs to change both these contributors to the obesity epidemic. Surveillance systems should be sensitive to the effects of these determinants on vulnerable groups, such as those experiencing socioeconomic deprivation and those in the very early stages of life. Disaggregated data by sex, ethnic group and social group should therefore be available.

A better understanding should be gained of the determinants of food consumption in different societal contexts and population groups, as well as of the determinants of dietary change in relation to the environmental factors affecting supply. Similarly, environmental factors that encourage greater physical activity must be further described.

The role of health protective factors – such as emotional resilience, mental health and social support – should be better described through case studies, among other things.

The dynamics of the food system, particularly in the expanding markets of eastern Europe, needs further exploration and the evolution of the food supply, particularly the price and availability of different products, needs consideration. The operation of the market could make a significant contribution to public health, if properly addressed by dealing with information asymmetry or external costs to society.

A system should be established for actively monitoring marketing practices in different European countries, particularly the advertising of food and non-alcoholic beverages to children.

3. The evidence base for interventions to counteract obesity

Main messages

- Standard evidence for successfully preventing obesity is hard to obtain. Randomized controlled trials are difficult to perform in open populations, and most controlled trials have been conducted in schools, health centres and workplaces, settings that offer the greatest opportunities for control and manipulation, thus creating a settings bias in the evidence base for policy-making.
- Interventions in the school, workplace and community have proven moderately effective in preventing obesity. Interventions in settings such as schools and preschool groups need to be integrated across food services, health education, physical education, play and sport, and should involve the participants in formulating policy.
- Micro-scale interventions are likely to have small effects unless supported by macro-scale interventions (for example, in food labelling, pricing and availability).
- Many cost-effective opportunities for promoting physical activity as a part of daily life exist across a range of settings, especially at the local and community levels. Promoting physical activity requires engaging different sectors, acquiring the capacity to gain their support and shifting from individual- to population-based interventions.
- Non-traditional evidence – including examples taken from other public health areas, modelling studies and expert committee recommendations – should also be considered to develop effective strategies for interventions that tackle the upstream determinants of health behaviour.
- Pricing strategies can influence purchasing behaviour, indicating that fiscal intervention is a plausible component of a policy to counter obesity. Taxation and pricing policies have contributed to preventing and controlling tobacco and alcohol consumption, although pricing policies for food or its main ingredients may be more complex to implement.

Introduction

Evidence on preventing obesity and on developing effective ways of improving dietary and physical activity patterns is growing rapidly. This chapter summarizes recent literature reviews and the recommendations of expert consultations. The evidence base for interventions at the individual, local and community levels (micro-interventions) is more developed than the evidence base for population-wide interventions (macro-interventions), such as regulations on food pricing or food promotion, although these have a greater potential to affect the whole population and depend less for their implementation on household or local community resources.

In striving to meet the criteria for the robust evidence that is expected in clinical trials, researchers have used settings for obesity intervention trials – such as schools and health centres – that can be controlled and manipulated to show the nature and extent of the effect of the intervention. However, this has created a settings bias in the evidence base. Other forms of evidence that do not depend on highly controlled settings need to be considered and included in assessing interventions.

In addition, care needs to be taken in defining the effect of interventions. Although some interventions measure their impact on the prevalence of obesity or on an indicator such as BMI, others have considered the effects of intervention on some behavioural determinant such as dietary choices or physical activity level. Measurement is difficult in all cases, and especially where it is based on self-assessment by participants.

The evidence can be drawn from experimental studies and from programme or policy evaluations, but it could also be extrapolated from modelling estimates (such as those used in economic analyses or in translating the effects of a programme to the whole population) or obtained from experience gained in tackling other public health issues (such as tobacco smoking) or from experience that scientists, practitioners and policy-makers have of the effects of certain policy measures on societal changes.

The conclusions of the chapter show that, although experimental evidence for an effective intervention strategy is lacking, many interventions show good potential for effectiveness. Sufficient evidence exists for immediate action, and continuing innovative approaches to prevention, adjusting local circumstances and conducting new research can improve the effectiveness of policies.

Interventions in micro-settings

There are three classical settings for intervention in health promotion: the health services (family services, specialist clinics and outreach health workers); schools and other social care facilities (for both educational and practical interventions); and the workplace (also for educational and practical interventions). Further settings include those that shape health behaviour, such as settings provided by economic operators (for example, shops and restaurants) targeting consumers, and by planners and designers (such as roads, parks and buildings) targeting users.

The most common settings for controlled trials are schools, where specific inputs (such as educational sessions, food services and physical activity sessions) can be measured and the experimental designs can ensure a degree of scientific validity to the results. Others suitable for controlled interventions include preschool community settings, health care facilities and workplaces.

The use of these settings, which are most amenable to controlled trials, has limited the information available to policy-makers and has led to concerns that evidence-based policy has too narrow a focus. Using their outcomes to determine policy poses serious problems: school, community and workplace interventions have been criticized for their lack of sustainability (few trials report long-term effects), lack of transferability and high levels of resources required. Further, most such interventions have had little or no effect in preventing overweight and only modest effects in altering the determinants of obesity, such as diet and physical activity patterns.

Family

A review in preparation suggests that interventions targeting children aged 2–5 years and their families and carers have equivocal effectiveness in helping to maintain a healthy weight or prevent overweight or obesity *(93)*. The studies suggest that small changes may be possible, and interventions are more likely to be effective if they focus specifically on preventing obesity (rather than changing diet and physical activity behaviours), and are intensive, costly, targeted and tailored to individual needs. The effectiveness of family interventions targeting older children is also equivocal. Family-based interventions may be less effective when trying to prevent obesity in adolescents.

Preschool and school

A review of the effectiveness of interventions to promote healthy eating in preschool settings for children aged 1–5 found that, while most studies demonstrated some positive effect on nutrition knowledge, the effect on eating behaviour was less frequently assessed and the results were inconsistent *(94)*. There were no data to evaluate long-term effectiveness on knowledge or behaviour.

There is strong evidence for obesity prevention in schools where the whole-school approach is adopted. Studies show that this approach can influence dietary intake through small but important changes in food choices made by children, such as an increase in fruit and vegetable intake, as well as an overall reduction in fat intake. Interestingly, girls are generally more responsive to a whole-class approach than boys. Breakfast clubs in schools show a beneficial effect on behaviour, dietary intake, health, social interaction, concentration and learning, attendance and punctuality. This can be of special importance, not only because obesity is more frequent in families of low socioeconomic status, but also because the effect can reach families whose members risk or are experiencing social exclusion.

Moderate evidence on helping children to maintain a healthy weight is found in school-based interventions that deliver an intense dietary education programme using multimedia (which, however, require significant additional financial and human resources). The same outcomes, though patchy, are shown by interventions focused on physical activity. Interventions that appear interesting and innovative to children (such as dance clubs), and those that aim to reduce television, videotape and video game use are also effective in helping maintain weight. In younger children, the most successful dietary interventions focus on only one aspect of a healthy diet such as fruit and vegetable intake, and use several approaches to promote the healthy eating messages, along with increased availability of relevant food. In older children, the factors that produce successful results are still less clear. Other moderate evidence on prevention of obesity in school is found in a comprehensive school policy on snacks brought to school, the presence of fruit tuck shops and walking and cycling to school.

Limited evidence is found for interventions based on the school fruit scheme, which can have a good impact in families from lower social grades. Limited evidence is also found for using tools such as presence of healthier options in food vending machines in schools.

Programmes to prevent obesity, especially for children and adolescents, should combine classic approaches to weight loss with enhancing self-esteem, developing healthy body-related attitudes, and ensuring that children do not engage in dysfunctional types of dieting associated to the development of eating disorders *(20)*. School prevention programmes should be comprehensive and ensure that the focus on obesity prevention does not increase the stigma associated with overweight or the risk of eating disorders *(95)*.

Workplace

Strategies that target adults at their place of work include a number of different approaches: nutrition education, prescription of aerobic or strength training exercise, training in behavioural techniques, the provision of self-help materials, prescription of specific diets and group or supervised exercise. Evidence of the effectiveness of workplace efforts to control overweight and obesity is not strong, but might encourage employers to provide such programmes. The literature supports an emphasis on interventions combining instruction in healthier eating with a structured approach to increasing physical activity in the workplace *(96)*. Workplace interventions on chronic disease and risk factor management have been successful in the United States, with an average return of 3.5 for health care cost savings and 5.8 for absenteeism savings *(97)*.

Community

Examples of more imaginative approaches used in community settings include:

- improved information and access to healthier food choices (for example, improving access to major stores and provision at local shops, establishing food cooperatives, community cafés, food-growing clubs);
- health promotion activities to improve knowledge and skills (for example, through shopping tours, cook-and-eat classes);
- improved provision and safety of walking and cycling routes; and
- local voucher schemes (for example, for local swimming pools).

Supermarket promotions appear to be effective in improving dietary intakes over the short term, particularly if accompanied by supporting information.

Table 2 shows examples of controlled trials of obesity prevention in children that have shown effectiveness. Interventions related to dietary change have been successful among younger children, using programmes that

Table 2. Examples of controlled, evaluated trials of obesity prevention among children

Country and intervention	Conclusion
Austria: PRESTO multiprofessional school educational intervention with children aged 10–12 years (pilot study) *(99)*	Improved nutritional knowledge, especially in higher-attainment students. No change in BMI.
Crete, Greece: school-based health education prospective study of children aged 6–12 years *(100,101)*	BMI improved in the intervention group compared with the control group, although BMI levels in both groups rose during the period, with increases in the proportion of children overweight.
Denmark: two-year intervention with family counselling, shopping and meal planning *(102)*	Children lost weight.
Germany: Kiel Obesity Prevention Study (KOPS), eight-year school-based intervention with children initially aged 5–7 years *(103)*	Improved nutrition knowledge and physical activity, reduced television viewing. Reduced adiposity indices (skinfold, percentage fat mass) versus controls.
Germany: StEP TWO school-based intervention with children aged 7–9 years *(104)*	Reduced rate of increase in BMI, reduced systolic blood pressure.
Israel: combined, structured multidisciplinary intervention with children and adolescents *(105)*	Decreased body weight, decreased BMI and improved fitness, especially if the parents were not overweight.
United Kingdom: "Be Smart": school and family intervention with children aged 5–7years *(106)*	Increased nutrition knowledge and fruit and vegetable intake. No significant change in overweight prevalence.
United Kingdom: "MAGIC": twelve-week programme (pilot study) to increase physical activity in preschool children aged 3–4 years *(107)*	Increased physical activity up to 40%. Unknown changes in adiposity.
United Kingdom: "APPLES": school-based intervention with children aged 7–11 years *(108,109)*	Some improvements in dietary patterns. No change in physical activity or BMI.

adopt the multimedia strategies used in marketing, such as videos, toys and cartoon characters, and with clearly defined positive and negative role models *(98)*.

Interventions in macro-settings

So far, policy responses have not been strong enough, have focused on single factors or have called on individual responsibility through educational campaigns. Several expert committees have agreed that elements of a successful intervention include a combination of policies and population-based programmes, regulation and action, part of a coordinated long-term public health strategy. Large-scale modifications of lifestyle are required and sufficient time should be allowed for the effects to take place.

Macroeconomic and whole-of-government interventions have been successfully performed for tobacco and alcohol, but less so in the area of nutrition. Therefore, not many examples can be analysed to assess effectiveness. Economic restructuring in Poland reduced animal fat consumption, promoted vegetable oil and increased fruit and vegetable consumption *(43)*. National demonstration programmes, such as that undertaken in Finland to reduce cardiovascular diseases, have shown the value of combining health education approaches (including multimedia campaigns) with structural changes such as pricing policies, agricultural support measures, food labelling and mass-catering interventions.

Several examples are available from outside Europe. In China, weight control, reduction of salt and alcohol intake and increased physical activity led to a decline in blood pressure in the framework of community-based programmes *(43)*.

Based on these suggestions, the target audiences for obesity interventions can be broadened to include food-processing industries (the food manufacturers, caterers and retailers that control much of what farmers produce and determine the quality of most of the food consumed), local governments, schools and workplaces, as well as the mass media, nongovernmental organizations, political pressure groups and legislators.

Promoting physical activity

As with the promotion of healthy diets, strategies to promote physical activity include not only the classical approaches, such as through leisure and sports facilities, schools, workplaces and health settings, but also transport and traffic planning and the design of buildings and urban environments.

Good evidence is available to show that school-based physical education with better-trained physical education teachers, comprehensive workplace approaches, prompts to increase stair use and the creation or improved access to places for physical activity, combined with informational outreach activities, can increase physical activity *(110)*. Good evidence also demonstrates that interventions that facilitate physically active transport, such as walking and cycling, raise levels of physical activity, and that perceived and objectively determined environmental attributes, such as aesthetics, convenience (sidewalks), access (green spaces), safety and security are associated with increased physical activity.

A combination of informational, behavioural, social, environmental and policy approaches might therefore prove effective in enhancing physical activity.

Economic instruments

Several authors have suggested that economic instruments may be used directly to affect food consumption patterns or physical activities. One approach is to apply negative economic incentives to obesity itself, such as by imposing higher health insurance costs for obese individuals. This would increase inequality in health and be highly unfair, considering the interpersonal variation in genetic predisposition to obesity. Another approach is to offer tax incentives, for example, to employers who offer nutrition counselling or physical activity facilities or to local authorities that build cycle routes and improve access to open spaces.

Specific taxation of energy-dense and nutrient-poor foods and subsidies for health promoting foods have also been considered. Good evidence shows that price manipulation affects consumption patterns and that this can be used to improve population dietary health, although care needs to be taken that price changes reduce socio-economic inequality, rather than increase it.

A longitudinal study of food prices and consumption in China found that increases in the prices of unhealthy foods were associated with decreased consumption of those foods *(111)*. In the United States, programmes to reduce the price of healthy foods led to a 78% increase in consumption *(43)*. Pricing is also recognized as a powerful influence on the purchasing of tobacco products and alcohol.

Modelling studies suggest that increasing the price of food components such as fat, saturated fat and sugar through fiscal measures instead of increasing the price of processed foods themselves, in combination with subsidies on fibre-rich foods, would reduce consumption of the taxed food components as well as total energy intake. Direct evidence from short-term studies conducted mainly in schools and workplaces has shown that reducing the price of fruits, vegetables and other healthy snacks increases the purchases of these foods and drinks *(74)*.

Even if imposing taxes or granting subsidies does not result in immediate behaviour change, it sends a strong message about the value of these foods and their impact on health – indeed, the threat of taxation may itself be a signal to commercial producers that they should review their product formulations. Investment companies have already warned leading food companies that they may be at commercial risk if they rely too heavily on a narrow range of energy-dense and nutrient-poor foods *(112)*.

Considering the context

The context in which interventions are implemented strongly determines their effectiveness. School food policies, for example, differ between schools that provide a meal service and those that do not, and between schools that charge a fee for meals and those that do not. Interventions to promote fruit and vegetable consumption may be ineffective if access to fresh fruit and vegetables is poor or their cost prohibitive. Interventions to increase bicycle use in cities where cycle lanes have been designed into the streets with traffic regulations that favour cyclists, such as in Copenhagen and Amsterdam, will differ from interventions in cities in which cycling is not supported by design or regulations.

Effective strategies to counter obesity need to consider cultural differences. In some cultures, high levels of obesity are acceptable, or even considered desirable, whereas other cultures have strong prejudice against overweight people, which may affect children as well as adults. In addition, not all cultures support physical activity of children in the same way, especially for girls. Further, care must be taken to ensure that programmes for preventing obesity do not induce unhealthy slimming practices or risky behaviour such as smoking to control weight. Measures to reduce the prevalence of obesity need to be introduced that emphasize healthy behaviour and activities, rather than idealized weight or appearance.

Some children and parents may resist the introduction of measures such as school policies that change the food environment. Analysis of best practices suggests that the targets for the interventions should be involved in planning them. A change in school practices, for example, might be most successful if all the relevant stakeholders – children, staff and parents – participate in the planning. This is especially important if their cooperation is needed for implementing the proposals. Such suggestions are consistent with the principles of the Ottawa and Bangkok charters for health promotion *(113,114)*.

Beyond the experimental evidence

In the absence of experimental evidence of success of interventions to prevent obesity, other forms of evidence may be considered.

Economic analyses may allow the extrapolation of evidence. Modelling estimates, for example, show that, in 20 years, nutrition labelling could produce health expenditure savings of US$ 1 billion in Australia, US$ 2.7 billion in the United States and US$ 5 billion in Canada *(43)*. A modelling study in Denmark of how households in different socioeconomic groups would respond to fluctuation in food prices showed that even small changes in value-added taxes could differentially improve the diet of poorer people *(115)*.

Parallel evidence (evidence applicable to other public health issues using similar strategies) supports regulatory approaches such as controls on marketing to children and mandatory clear nutritional food labelling. Such approaches have proved valuable in controlling exposure to tobacco smoke, promoting the use of car seat-belts, restricting the promotion of breast-milk substitutes and limiting alcohol consumption among young people.

Expert opinion also provides useful guidance. It can consider target groups, settings and approaches that are not amenable to controlled trials but that, based on other forms of evidence, are considered to be important in reducing the risk of obesity in the population. WHO expert consultations *(1,75)* recommended measures to prevent overweight and obesity, and indicated the need to consider population-based interventions and to tackle the underlying determinants of food choices and physical activity levels, instead of simply assuming that individuals should improve their diets and physical activity levels.

Several initiatives are not being undertaken in scientifically controlled settings, but show what is feasible and politically acceptable and may be considered worth adopting before waiting for a full evaluation. Table 3 shows examples.

Building evidence for effective interventions: the next steps

New methods for evaluating evidence and assessing cost–effectiveness need to be developed to support the selection of interventions. Cost estimates will need to be based on information on the resource requirements for interventions.

Policies need to be developed that acknowledge the limitations of traditional approaches to evidence, acknowledge that public health interventions will involve risk (uncertainty of outcome) and accept that levels of return

Table 3. Examples of novel interventions, policies and practices in Europe that may help prevent obesity

Country	Interventions or policies
Denmark	6-a-day programme *(116)*: increased fruit consumption in the workplace and at school
France	Tax on television commercials for soft drinks Ban on vending machines in all schools
Germany	Monitoring authority for commercial material in schools
Greece	Fast-food chains prohibited from running school food shops or canteens
Greece and Scotland, United Kingdom	Nutrition standards for school meals
Ireland, Sweden	Controls on television advertising targeting children
Kazakhstan	Network of Health Promoting Schools *(117)*: 300 participating schools
Norway	Maternal leave to promote breastfeeding *(118)* (98% of women leave hospital maternity wards breastfeeding; 90% are breastfeeding at 3–4 months; 75% of women are still breastfeeding at 6 months)
Russian Federation	Growing vegetables on rooftops *(119)*: about 15 rooftop gardens in St Petersburg contribute significantly to fruit and vegetable supplies for local communities in low-income areas
Sweden	Provision of free school meals following voluntary guidelines
Switzerland	Companies give advice to employees about their children's excess weight
United Kingdom	Water is Cool in School *(120)*: several schools have installed water coolers and offer free water bottles for every child in the school, which has helped to reduce disruptions to lessons and increases concentration School walking buses *(121)*: adults accompany children in a group walking to school along a set route, picking up additional passengers along the way Fighting Fat, Fighting Fit, a television campaign directed at the whole population *(122)*: good awareness ratings, but recall of the lifestyle message was poorer among those with lower levels of education and among ethnic minority groups, and participation was low, even among target groups Eating fruit and vegetables will help get a school swimming pool Replacement of vending machines with school milk bar Subsidized use of sports centres for local schools Children leaving schools in cars must wait 10 minutes before leaving Sales tax on "luxury" foods

(effects of intervention) will vary. For example, there is insufficient direct, robust evidence to introduce controls on the marketing of energy-dense and nutrient-poor foods to children or to intervene in markets using fiscal measures to change consumption patterns, but there are sufficient indications to believe that these measures offer great potential as part of a portfolio of options to counter obesity and encourage better health.

Since policy-makers may choose to implement economic or other social policy instruments in the absence of conclusive evidence, these interventions should be subject to prospective, ongoing evaluation. Evaluations of economic instruments should include both their impact on the consumption of specific foods and their ability to shift the balance of energy intake and expenditure.

The policy environment can influence active living through a variety of mechanisms. Some are domain specific, as in the case of budgets for transport and traffic management or urban planning and housing policies. Others are cross cutting, as in health care policies that provide incentives and counselling for physical activity. Innovative interventions and approaches that have proven effective in other sociocultural contexts should be documented.

4. Management and treatment of obesity

Main messages

- In adults, high-quality evidence supports the effectiveness of low-energy diets for treating obesity. Restricting dietary fat appears to be an effective method of lowering energy density and is associated with spontaneous weight loss.
- High-quality evidence indicates that increased physical activity is effective in maintaining a modest total weight loss and provides additional health benefits. However, diet alone appears to be more effective than exercise alone in losing weight.
- No evidence to date confirms effectiveness beyond two years or confirms longer-term benefit against associated health risks.
- Treating associated health risks and established complications is as important as managing obesity.
- Children can achieve several benefits through dietary control, but several negative consequences may also arise unless precautions are taken, including loss of lean body mass, reduced linear growth and exacerbation of eating disorders. Weight maintenance regimes (with nutritional counselling) are preferred for all but very obese children until after puberty. For very obese children or moderately obese children with additional complications, a balanced low-energy diet using normally available foods is recommended.
- Reducing inactivity, increasing walking and developing an activity programme can increase the effectiveness of obesity therapy and, even when these do not reduce obesity, they can independently reduce morbidity.
- Parental involvement in treatment programmes is necessary for successful weight loss both among young children and, to a lesser extent, among adolescents.

Introduction

The earlier chapters focus on the need for policies and population-wide interventions to prevent obesity.

This chapter turns to the principles of treating obesity. Since increased morbidity risk is already present in pre-obese individuals, weight reduction should be advised even in the case of moderately excess body weight, in order to prevent further progression to more pronounced forms of overweight.

Interventions leading to weight loss in adults can show rapid benefit. For example, weight loss in women results in a reduction of mortality in the first two years, and there are additional improvements in risk factors for poor health and complications from other diseases. However, successful weight loss among both adults and children requires resources and the working time of multiple professions and, even then, successful, sustained weight loss can be difficult to achieve.

Weight loss should not be the only objective for treating obesity. Additional aims are to reduce the risk to health and the complications from associated disease that may be present. Further, clinicians and patients should be aware that treatment is not just for the short term but should be sustained.

Screening of population groups can be considered if effective follow-up services are available and accessible, preferably if in the context of assessment of multiple risk factors for noncommunicable diseases.

Intervention approaches: adults

Mild to moderate weight loss in adults can be achieved and maintained by lifestyle interventions. Primary care doctors, provided they have received specific training, have a role in counselling on diet and physical activity for pre-obese conditions. Specialized centres are better placed to deliver counselling and monitoring for more severe conditions.

Dietary treatment

High-quality evidence supports the effectiveness of low-energy diets for treating obesity. Restricting dietary fat appears to be an effective method of lowering energy density and is associated with spontaneous weight loss.

Modest reductions in energy intake (about 2.5 MJ (600 kcal) per day) may improve compliance, and this has been recommended as a dietary option for weight management. Evidence also indicates that low-fat diets combined with energy restriction and low-fat diets alone are effective long-term interventions. Very-low-energy diets are effective for acute weight loss, but are generally reserved for people with severe obesity (BMI ≥35) and associated illnesses that justify rapid weight loss. Evidence suggests that these diets are no more effective in long-term management than more moderate dietary strategies.

Several unbalanced dietary regimens are advised by some health practitioners, often not adequately qualified, or even through the media. This practice should be discouraged, particularly if prolonged, as it can lead to poor coverage of nutrient needs.

Physical activity

High-quality evidence shows that increased physical activity is effective in maintaining a modest total weight loss. However, diet alone appears to be more effective than exercise alone. Physical activity on prescription by primary care doctors has been advised in some countries.

Behavioural therapy

A combination of behavioural therapy techniques in conjunction with other weight loss approaches is effective over a one-year period. There is limited evidence for the effectiveness of extending behavioural therapy beyond this period.

Pharmaceutical treatment

Anti-obesity drugs are effective in increasing the proportion of people achieving modest weight loss for up to two years, but they have to be combined with dietary treatment and have side effects. Modest evidence confirms effectiveness beyond this period, and little evidence confirms long-term reduction of disability and death. The United Kingdom's National Institute for Clinical Excellence has issued technological guidelines on sibutramine *(123)* and orlistat *(124)*, two of the most popular drugs. Different countries have taken different approaches on making these medicines available through their reimbursement systems.

Surgery

Obesity surgery is the only proven intervention to maintain weight reduction in severely obese patients for the longer term (more than 10 years). This weight reduction is associated with significant metabolic benefits, especially a reduction in the incidence of type 2 diabetes.

Surgery is effective for the treatment of obesity when all other non-surgical methods have failed. It is, however, a very expensive intervention, and carries a 0.5% mortality risk. The development of any service requires adequately trained multidisciplinary teams to operate and provide long-term support.

Treatment of associated health conditions

Obesity co-morbidities have to be considered, and screening for other risk factors, such as alcohol or smoking, should also be performed. Treatment of overweight and obesity, which requires appropriately trained health professionals, not only necessitates losing weight but also managing the associated health complications. Treating associated health risks and established complications is as important as managing obesity. Too often the treatment of risks or complications is delayed in the mistaken belief that weight reduction will achieve sufficient benefit. Binge eating, along with presence of a mental disorder, has been associated with poor treatment outcome of obesity *(20)*; health and mental health professionals should be aware of this and screen for mental disorders even if they are not suggested by the initial complaint *(20,21)*.

Intervention approaches: children and adolescents

Reviews of the treatment of obesity among children and adolescents have shown that, when weight is reduced, several associated factors also improve, but successful, sustained weight reduction is hard to achieve. Approaches for children and adolescents are generally designed to limit further weight gain and to manage and alleviate the associated illnesses.

Motivation is essential: if the child or an influential parent is not motivated, then the prospects for successful intervention are poor. Practitioners may need to make themselves familiar with techniques for gaining and increasing motivation among children and their families.

Compared with younger children, adolescents are less likely to accept a highly controlled home or school regimen; their dropout rate is higher and they have a wider range of strategies for avoiding treatment and inaccurate self-reporting. Adolescents are in danger of falling in the gap between paediatric and adult services, refusing to be treated "like children" and failing to attend appointments. New strategies – such as those involving communication through the Internet, better involvement of adolescents in designing their own management programmes and peer support strategies – need to be explored.

Dietary treatment

Dietary control can provide several benefits, but several negative consequences may also arise, including loss of lean body mass, reduced linear growth and exacerbation of eating disorders. Weight maintenance regimes (with nutritional counselling) are preferred for all but very obese children until after puberty. For very obese children or moderately obese children with additional complications, a balanced low-energy diet using normally available foods is recommended.

Physical activity

Reducing inactivity, increasing walking and developing an activity programme can increase the effectiveness of obesity therapy and, even when these do not reduce obesity, they can independently reduce morbidity. Strategies for raising energy expenditure involve increasing physical activity and, as a separate strategy, reducing sedentary behaviour such as television watching. Simple measures such as reducing children's television and the use of videotapes and video games can significantly contribute to decreasing overweight in children.

The type of exercise used (exercise that is part of daily life involving games, swimming, sports, dance and cycling versus programmed aerobic exercise) also appears to be important for sustained weight loss. Both forms help promote weight loss in the initial phase, but children and adolescents are more likely to continue in the long term with exercise that is integrated into daily life. Physicians can prescribe physical activity, as well as other forms of treatment.

Psychological and familial support

The family influences the child's food and activity habits, and any effective treatment must take this into account. Parental involvement in treatment programmes is necessary for successful weight loss among both young children and, to a lesser extent, adolescents. Clinicians should note potential barriers to parental involvement in treating children. In some families, for cultural or psychological reasons, parents may not perceive the child to be obese. In other families, parents may acknowledge that the child is obese but deny that this is of any consequence.

Behavioural and psychological forms of therapy that help to enhance physical activity and healthy eating habits are considered valuable for the long-term success of treatment among obese children and adolescents. With preschool children, group teaching is more important than individual treatment, and the whole family should be involved. By the time children reach puberty, they are creating their own groups and social networks, and individual treatment may be more appropriate. Forms of treatment can include cognitive behavioural therapy, family therapy, specialized schools and hospital treatment, especially if they also suffer from co-morbid mental health problems, whether as a cause or consequence, and there is evidence of some effectiveness of behavioural and psychoeducative approaches *(125–127)*.

Residential treatment

In some circumstances, interventions may be considered more effective if delivered in a more controlled environment, using a programmed combination of therapeutic measures to tackle the range of health effects of obesity. Residential programmes are best reserved for older children who can accept residing away from the family home and can form social networks with peers undergoing the programme.

Pharmaceutical treatment

Several drug therapies for adults have been considered for adolescents, but most of these have yet to reach approval stage. Until more extensive safety and efficacy data are available, medication for weight loss should be used only on an experimental basis in adolescents and children.

Surgery

Surgical interventions are not yet recommended for use among children and adolescents with common forms of obesity. The safety and effectiveness of surgical treatments have not been sufficiently established in these patient groups, and other approaches should be tried first. Surgery should be considered only when all else has failed, when children have achieved adult height and when severe, potentially life-threatening complications of obesity are present.

Management and treatment: the next steps

Lifestyle counselling in health care with respect to diet and physical activity can reduce body weight at reasonable cost. A recent review indicated that a weight loss of 5% after one year can be achieved at a cost of around €150 per patient *(128)*.

Few health care professionals have been taught about nutrition and physical activity or realistic weight loss goals, and obesity treatment is frequently instituted without the benefit of an integrated programme for managing lifestyle. There is thus considerable scope for developing better training for the professionals responsible for treating obese people or providing support services: clinicians, family counsellors, physical activity specialists, dieticians and practice managers, who may need to coordinate home-based interventions.

Childhood obesity screening can be of value when the screened obese individuals are ready to have further assessment and to make changes to achieve a healthy weight; when further assessment or other necessary treatment facilities are available in the community; and when effective intervention programmes and follow-up activities for the identified children are accessible and available.

Health systems need to cope with huge numbers of overweight children and adults, who present not only with overweight but also with related disorders such as type 2 diabetes and coronary heart disease. Health ministries and professional organizations should therefore consider the challenge of how best to cope with such large numbers of people who might benefit from health care assessment and management. Physicians often consider themselves already overwhelmed by the clinical load, so novel approaches need to be considered in using other health care personnel in assessing, managing and following up. Further, specialized services providing treatment and staffed with multidisciplinary teams should have adequate territorial distribution and acceptable waiting times. This is a major challenge that no national health system has yet tackled successfully and coherently.

5. Development of policies to counteract obesity

Main messages

- Countries have made progress in raising awareness and an increasing number have launched policies and action plans in recent years, but no country has yet effectively managed to bring the obesity epidemic under control.
- Countries and international organizations urgently need to increase investment in preventing obesity. Children, young people and groups with low socioeconomic status are priority groups. Women have to be given special attention in view of the importance of metabolic imprinting and their role as care providers, as well as their vulnerability at certain life stages.
- A review of country policy statements found good awareness of the need for a wide portfolio of policy options involving several sectors and a range of stakeholders.
- Health ministries should recognize that other sectors have provided the main drivers of the obesity epidemic. Health ministries therefore need to provide the necessary leadership and stewardship to ensure that all stakeholders contribute to the overall national efforts to improve diets and physical activity levels for preventing obesity.
- Health and economic assessment is needed in each country to illustrate the dimensions of the problem and to mobilize multisectoral commitment. Consensus has to be reached within the government and its ministries about the importance of the problem, its determinants and the joint responsibility for improving the situation.
- Each ministry that has an influence on the determinants of obesity needs to interact with a wide range of private, public and civil stakeholders at the national, regional and local levels to formulate measures that can be applied in practice.
- An investment approach that acknowledges risk (uncertainty of outcome) and allows for different levels of return (effects of intervention) provides a useful model for policy-making.
- Action to promote the demand for and supply of healthier food includes: developing and improving national food-based dietary guidelines; implementing measures to regulate prices, to impose food standards and to support socially disadvantaged groups in accessing healthy foods; reducing the market pressure on children by regulating advertising and obtaining cooperation from the mass media and Internet providers; conducting nutrition education and improving labelling schemes; promoting breastfeeding; improving nutrition profiles of foods by reducing their content of sugar, salt and saturated fat; avoiding production incentives for fat, sugar and alcohol and promoting the cultivation and marketing of fruits and vegetables; providing healthy food in schools; and improving catering, including in workplaces.
- Action to promote physical activity in the population includes: enhancing the affordability of and access to places and facilities for physical activity; promoting safe physically active transport, especially for commuting to schools and workplaces; adapting workplaces to improve the motivation for being physically active; stimulating changes in the urban environment to promote physical activity; communicating with the public; improving school physical activity programmes; promoting physically active recreation and promoting individual counselling via health professionals.
- Health impact assessment is a valuable tool to encourage intersectoral policies for preventing obesity.
- Involving multiple stakeholders is a crucial component of developing new strategies for tackling the prevention and management challenges of obesity. Stakeholders from outside the health sector can play a key role in reorienting public health policies.

- Not all stakeholders share a fundamental commitment to health goals. Therefore, more effective ways and arguments are needed to win the support of other sectors by making them more aware of the role they can play and what they can gain from facilitating and promoting healthy diets and physical activity. The stakeholder approach can be strengthened by proposals to legislate or regulate rather than relying on voluntary participation alone, as this will create a level playing field for economic operators.
- Nongovernmental organizations and professional bodies can offer valuable support for policies and can provide networking and other services to promote and monitor policies.
- Monitoring and evaluation is an essential tool to assess the progress of policies and provide an opportunity for review. Sufficient means and time need to be ensured for well-conducted evaluations and the body responsible for monitoring and evaluation should be independent of political and commercial interests.
- International action is essential to support national policies.

Introduction

Countries have made progress in raising awareness and an increasing number have launched policies and action plans in recent years, but none has yet succeeded in breaking the trend of increasing obesity rates. The rapid proliferation of the problem requires inventive solutions as well as inventive structures. This chapter considers the principles of strategies for preventing obesity and the various stakeholders involved in the process of forming and implementing policy.

Earlier chapters have emphasized the need to consider a range of policies, involving an assortment of stakeholders across many sectors, to counter obesity at the population as well as individual level. A portfolio of investments relevant to the national and local culture and to the regulatory context is recommended.

To improve dietary habits and increase physical activity, measures should primarily be directed at the level in society where conditions for healthy dietary habits and physical activity are created, thus making adopting a healthy lifestyle easy. Experience has shown that people make healthy choices more often if the surrounding environment is supportive. Health promotion directed exclusively at the individual, without affecting the societal conditions for health, does not achieve the desired effects and may increase inequality in health. Stakeholders also need to be involved in implementing policies, and their participation in developing policy can provide valuable political support. Further, areas of greatest need and with optimal potential health gain, such as socially disadvantaged communities and young people, should be prioritized.

This approach has been identified in the WHO Global Strategy on Diet, Physical Activity and Health (adopted in 2002 in World Health Assembly resolution WHA55.23) and in regional initiatives such as the EU Platform on Diet, Physical Activity and Health and the present WHO European initiative on counteracting obesity.

An investment portfolio approach is needed, involving a set of policy measures across different sectors and at different levels, taking cultural and economic contexts into account.

The results of policy implementation need to be evaluated, and this requires continuous monitoring of the indicators of obesity and its determinants, such as dietary patterns and physical activity levels. The results of the monitoring need to be used as the basis for regular reviews of policy instruments and their implementation. Such policy reviews should be undertaken by bodies that are independent of commercial and political interests, such as an independent obesity observatory, nutrition council or public health institute, with a mandate to make policy recommendations.

Existing international action frameworks

Several recent international policy instruments have addressed the most important risk factors for obesity: unhealthy diets and physical inactivity.

The **WHO Global Strategy on Diet, Physical Activity and Health** *(129)* is a set of policy options addressed to governments and other stakeholders. The technical recommendations are based on a robust body of evidence from a variety of scientific sources, and the policy recommendations were developed on the basis of political, financial, health infrastructure, workforce and other practical considerations. The aim is that countries and other stakeholders should decide on the policy options that best fit their local circumstances. Despite compelling evidence on the rapid growth of the epidemic of noncommunicable diseases and their common risk factors in all parts of the world (except sub-Saharan Africa), investment by governments and international agencies to reduce them is well below what is required. European countries are generally more willing to act than countries in other parts of the world. However, the proportion of total burden from noncommunicable diseases in the European Region is the highest in the world, so countries in the European Region need to do far more.

Some improvements are noted in national capacity and capability to prevent and control noncommunicable diseases and their common risk factors. Compared with the global assessment in 2000–2001, more countries now have capacity to develop policies, plans and programmes for preventing and controlling noncommunicable diseases, and several have developed specific responses to the request made in connection with the WHO Global Strategy on Diet, Physical Activity and Health. However, many countries have not developed appropriate national responses to the problems caused by noncommunicable diseases, or responded to the recommendations made by the Global Strategy.

Some changes have taken place in the private sector in response to the development and adoption of the Global Strategy. Manufacturers of food and non-alcoholic beverages have been active in developing new and healthier product options and improving consumer information about their products. These actions are encouraging but remain ad hoc and limited in scope, and further industry-wide action needs to be applied to mainstream commercial food and drink products. Nongovernmental and professional organizations can significantly influence the implementation of the objectives of the Global Strategy, and excellent working relationships have been established with these groups.

The Codex Alimentarius Commission, the joint standard-setting body for trade in food of WHO and the Food and Agriculture Organization of the United Nations (FAO), has taken steps to use its remit to support the Global Strategy. Its remit includes labelling and health claims as well as food composition and ingredient specifications, and the Commission is considering how it can use its powers to enhance consumers' ability to make healthy choices.

The **EU Platform on Diet, Physical Activity and Health** *(130)* was established in 2005 as a forum involving stakeholders from commercial, professional, consumer and other civil-society organizations, coordinated by the European Commission. The Platform has held a series of meetings and workshops and has elicited a range of commitments from stakeholder participants that are being monitored and evaluated. A review of the Platform is anticipated in 2007. The Commission's activities have been supported by the European Economic and Social Committee, a consultative body consisting of economic operators, labour representatives and civil-society organizations, which has also issued its own opinion on the need to tackle obesity across all sectors. After the Platform was launched, the European Commission issued a green paper on the promotion of healthy diets and physical activity as part of a public consultation on how to reduce obesity and the prevalence of associated noncommunicable diseases in the EU. The green paper called for concrete suggestions and ideas on action that can be taken in all sectors and at every level of society to address this serious problem and to encourage Europeans towards healthier lifestyles. The European Commission intends to publish a report in early 2007 on the outcome of the consultation, proposing action on nutrition and physical activity.

The **European Strategy for the Prevention and Control of Noncommunicable Diseases** *(131)* in the WHO European Region, approved by the WHO Regional Committee for Europe in September 2006, advocates a comprehensive strategy that simultaneously promotes population-level health promotion and disease prevention programmes, actively targets individuals at high risk, and maximizes population coverage of effective treatments and integrated action on risk factors and their underlying determinants across sectors, combined with efforts to strengthen health systems towards improved prevention and control.

The WHO **Global Strategy for Infant and Young Child Feeding** *(132)* advocates exclusive breastfeeding up to 6 months of age, followed by timely introduction of adequate and safe complementary foods. The proven connection between infant feeding and early development of obesity makes the implementation of this strategy particularly important. The European Commission has also published a **Blueprint for Action on the Promotion of Breastfeeding in Europe**, in recognition of the evidence that breastfeeding reduces children's risk of infections, may decrease the risk of later obesity and has beneficial effects "for mothers, families, the community, the health and social system, the environment and the society in general" *(133)*.

The **European strategy for child and adolescent health and development** *(134)*, approved by the WHO Regional Committee for Europe in September 2005, specifically prioritizes good nutrition as a basis for healthy development and highlights the need to prevent obesity in school-aged children, through action in different sectors.

The **Children's Environment and Health Action Plan for Europe** (CEHAPE) *(135)*, approved in 2004, commits the countries in the European Region to pursuing a decrease in morbidity from lack of adequate physical activity by promoting safe, secure and supporting human settlements for all children. In particular, it advocates road safety measures, child-friendly urban planning and, safe and accessible facilities for social interaction, play and sports.

The **transport, health and environment pan-European programme** (THE PEP) *(136)*, adopted in 2002, commits countries to developing measures for promoting and improving safe conditions for cycling and walking, with particular reference to children.

Current national policies on obesity in countries of the European Region

Most countries in the WHO European Region have developed nutrition action plans or public health strategies dealing with obesity risk factors, while only a few are dealing with physical activity. A comprehensive assessment of the policy developments on nutrition, physical activity and the prevention of obesity is given in a specific background paper for the Ministerial Conference on Obesity *(137)*. An integrated analysis of this assessment is provided here.

- The diffusion of **policy documents** concerned with food and nutrition is high in the European Region, although their main focus is not always nutrition, but may be physical activity, cardiovascular disease prevention, public health, sustainable development or environmental health. Obesity prevention is tackled within a specific obesity action plan in the cases of Denmark, Ireland, Portugal, Slovakia and Spain, or as part of a nutrition action plan or a public health strategy. Estonia, Finland, the Netherlands, Norway, Slovakia, Slovenia and the United Kingdom have each developed an additional separate national policy document dealing with physical activity. In the Russian Federation, the development of such an action plan is under consideration.
- Strategies in Armenia, Azerbaijan, Georgia, Kazakhstan, Kyrgyzstan, the Republic of Moldova, Ukraine and Tajikistan, for instance, focus strongly on nutrition and food safety within national documents or separate projects such as micronutrient deficiency prevention and breastfeeding promotion. Promotion of physical activity and prevention of obesity are often part of those strategies.
- Besides making a statement of general objectives, many countries set specific **numeric dietary goals**, but few have defined quantifiable goals for overweight and obesity and physical activity. The United Kingdom, for example, has set a goal of no further increase in the prevalence of obesity among children younger than 11 years by 2010. Bulgaria and France aim to reduce the number of overweight and obese people by 10% and 20%, respectively.
- Most strategies identify stakeholders, and measures to involve them include creating **partnerships**, networks or platforms or achieving commitment through signed agreements. Examples of those activities are Germany's Platform for Diet and Physical Activity, Poland's Platform for Action on Diet, Physical Activity and Health, the Dutch Covenant on Overweight and Obesity, Estonia's Health Promoting Networks, Switzerland's

Network Health and Physical Activity, Armenia's Interministerial Commission and several public–private partnerships on the national or local level, as in Denmark, Greece and the United Kingdom.

- Specific policy **actions** in multiple settings (schools, workplaces, health care services), on multiple levels (national, regional, local level) and in multiple sectors (environment, agriculture, sport, research, housing) have been developed in Denmark, Finland, Ireland, Italy, Norway, Spain, Sweden and the United Kingdom.
- Most countries have an **institutional structure**, such as a food and nutrition council or an institute for public health with various responsibilities, ranging from technical support to advising, planning and implementing the strategies. Some countries established a specific obesity institution for policy development, such as the Czech National Council for Obesity, the Danish Association for the Study of Obesity, the Portuguese Society for the Study of Obesity and the taskforces on obesity in Ireland and Israel. In some countries, especially the Nordic countries, policy councils have a long history. Recent examples of newly created institutions that are responsible for advice and better coordination between sectors are an advisory body in Estonia, the Nutrition Council in Latvia, the Centre for Nutrition, and Diet in The former Yugoslav Republic of Macedonia and the Food and Nutrition Committee in Turkey. These may have a limited lifespan (as the Taskforce in Ireland) or operate on a continuing basis (as the Obesity Observatory in Spain).
- All policy strategies identify **target groups** according to the life-course approach. Other target groups include people who have low socioeconomic status or limited education, or are distressed, chronically ill, disabled, members of ethnic minority groups or immigrants.
- **Schools** are the settings where most interventions take place, with the common goal of changing the school environment by providing a good framework for physical activity and strengthening health education. In Malta, a specific taskforce is working on a national policy on healthy school nutrition environments. In Spain, an initiative is addressing the school environment and the whole-school approach has been introduced in Croatia. In Belgium, the Flemish Community is currently developing a strategic and operational plan for the educational sector. Many countries aim at improving school food in canteens or through catering, as in the case of Hungary and the Netherlands, with a national school canteen programme, and Estonia, where free school meals will be provided to schoolchildren from first to ninth grades and in vocational schools. In Norway, a project on physical activity and healthy meals was recently introduced to disseminate good models and advise local school authorities on key factors of success. Vending machines are a controversial subject of national interventions, which aim either to eliminate them or to optimize their content. In France, for instance, a law was introduced to ban vending machines from schools. France, Latvia, the Netherlands, Norway and the United Kingdom attempt to provide fruit free of charge or make it easily accessible in schools.
- Actions in the **workplace** setting include flexible working hours, reduced rates for gym membership, incentives for cycling or walking to work, access to showers and changing facilities, promotion and information on healthy nutrition and lifestyle and optimizing workplace canteens. To promote cycling to and from the workplace, Austria and Sweden started competitive initiatives between companies. In Norway, a new working environment act obliges employers to consider physical activity as a part of their responsibility.
- Some policy documents consider **capacity building**, including the need to train health workers, teachers in food, nutrition and physical education, child-care workers and other deliverers of health promotion strategies and to provide training for the inspection of services, such as schools and child-care centres, where health policies are required to be implemented. Ireland suggests that programmes be developed to educate and train health professionals in the appropriate and sensitive management of overweight and obesity. Denmark emphasizes the need for psychological insight and practical knowledge. The Norwegian Action Plan on Physical Activity proposes introducing health impact assessment in the medical curriculum.
- In **urban planning**, most countries focus on active transport with, for instance, the construction of safe walking and cycling paths. The Czech Republic, Denmark, Finland, France, Germany, Norway and the United Kingdom all have national cycling strategies. Initiatives to discourage the use of cars and encourage children to walk to school, such as walking buses, have been promoted in Italy, Malta and the United Kingdom. In Malta, a

transport and environment committee was created to promote safe transport, including walking and cycling to school. The Finnish "Jaloin project" focuses on pedestrian and cycling traffic. In the United Kingdom, a action plan called Travelling to School outlines a series of measures through which national and local government and schools can promote more walking, cycling and bus use on the journey to and from school.

- Examples of mass events, where the whole population is motivated to engage in some sort of physical activity on a specific day, have taken place in Kazakhstan and Switzerland.
- **Housing policy** measures are part of Sweden's effort to create environments that support a physically active life, as part of the proposed action plan for healthy dietary habits and increased physical activity. In Norway, a planning and building act is being revised to create more activity-enhancing surroundings.
- There are several examples of projects on both national and local levels: Belgium, the Russian Federation and the United Kingdom, for instance, have regional policies and programmes in addition to their national strategies.
- Several countries use or are considering adopting **fiscal measures**, such as taxing unhealthy foods and providing incentives to encourage the supply and consumption of healthy foods or access to physical activity, but the purpose is more often to raise revenue rather than promote health. Norway's document specifically suggests lowering the prices of fruits and vegetables and subsidizing their distribution to remote areas as well as raising taxes on energy-dense and nutrient-poor foods. In Switzerland, a proposal on the taxation of energy-dense foods was recently presented, but will not be implemented at present.
- In several countries, a dialogue has begun with the food industry on a revision of **food product design**. The Government of the United Kingdom is aiming to reduce salt, added sugar and fat in processed food and will further develop and publish guidance on portion sizes. In the Czech Republic, a technology platform has been established by the Federation of the Food and Drink Industries and, in Greece, a platform is currently being developed for successful collaboration between the food industry and the Ministry of Health.
- Most countries are considering changes in **food labelling**, and there is a trend towards improved information and easily understood labels. Some examples of easily understood markings are Sweden's keyhole symbol on food labels, identifying foods low in fat, sugar or salt or high in dietary fibre, and the United Kingdom's traffic-light system, marking products with a red, amber or green light to show whether their levels of fat, saturated fat, sugar and salt content are high, medium or low, respectively.
- **Marketing food and beverages to children** is a major issue in the European Region. Some countries, such as Sweden and Norway, have introduced statutory regulations that ban this form of advertisement, and non-statutory guidelines that impose some limitations exist in Finland and Ireland. Other countries, such as the Netherlands, Portugal and Spain, rely on self-regulation, established by organizations set up by the advertising and media industries. In France, all television advertising and other forms of marketing of processed foods and foods or drinks containing added fats, sweeteners and salt must be accompanied by a health warning on the principles of dietary education as approved by National Institute of Health Education; alternatively the advertiser must contribute a tax (1.5% of the annual expenditure on that advertisement) to the funding of nutritional information and education campaigns.

In conclusion, country policies recognize the importance of an environmental approach to improving health, the need to act at the national, community and individual levels and the need to involve stakeholders in implementing policy. Clear and realistic objectives and setting priorities among the suggested actions are necessary for successfully implementing policy and evaluating the outcome. Experiences and examples of successful interventions on a large scale need to be exchanged, and collaboration between and harmonization of national activities need to be strengthened.

Development of strategies and action plans

Governments have a managing role in developing, implementing and monitoring an obesity prevention strategy. As indicated earlier, the determinants of obesity risk lie across a broad range of sectors and ministerial responsibilities, and health ministries need to collaborate with colleagues in other ministries to achieve a comprehensive strategy for addressing obesity.

A strategy to counter obesity can be part of general public health documents (such as noncommunicable disease strategies) or a food, nutrition and lifestyle action plan, or it can be an independent document that makes cross-references to the related strategies and plans for diet and physical activity.

The ministry of health may take the leadership in the development of the strategy, identify relevant policy areas and call for the establishment of an intersectoral group or committee including the actors required to develop a multisectoral approach, in collaboration with technical experts and other relevant informants. This role can be effectively performed through specialized national agencies.

In the preparation phase, the ministry of health could provide factual information about diet, physical activity and obesity in the population through:

- the establishment of monitoring systems for diet, physical activity and obesity;
- national goals for diet, physical activity and obesity;
- analyses of underlying determinants of dietary habits and physical activity;
- analyses of existing obesity, nutrition, noncommunicable disease and other public health plans to identify areas of weakness and of strength and opportunities for consolidation and expansion; and
- the use of health impact assessment methods.

Other ministries and agencies identified could analyse existing policies in their respective sectors and evaluate their impact on health and nutritional status.

In the strategy design phase, the health and other ministries could formulate measures for tackling the existing obesogenic factors within their respective policy areas. Each ministry and agency could develop a set of measures for implementation within its area, including the revision of existing policies. The intersectoral group or committee could prepare the draft plan and consult with local communities, the private sector and nongovernmental organizations. Suggested measures should be concrete, and the actors responsible for implementation need to be identified and their participation confirmed. Issues such as financing of implementation need to be considered and the financing assured. Policy decisions will be made on the basis of the expected effectiveness of the solutions, their potential side effects, the feasibility of implementation, cost, sustainability and acceptability to stakeholders.

An investment approach to health promotion

The fact that the evidence base for interventions is limited and subject to a settings bias is a strong argument for looking beyond the classical medical paradigm that depends on controlled trials and instead considering an alternative paradigm – the investment portfolio – which derives from banking and financial risk management.

In this approach, interventions are defined as investments, and an investment portfolio should carry a mixture of safe, low-return interventions and risky but potentially high-return interventions. Risk can be estimated based on the consistency of the impact of an intervention and indications of its likely effectiveness. Thus, intensive interventions within small groups or individuals might be classified as low-risk and low-return, as they consistently result in changes in behaviour but with only a small effect on the prevalence of obesity in the population *(138,139)*.

In health promotion, a return on investment can be measured in terms of expected health gains and other desired outcomes. The risk can be measured according to the consistency of the impact of an intervention across different population groups, its penetration within a given population group and indications of its likely effectiveness. The risk also includes the resources likely to be used. These need to be based on estimates of the resources needed to undertake an intervention – and the published literature has a surprising lack of such information.

Investments in health can also be conceptualized in terms of a projection table in which the return on investment is displayed in two dimensions: population impact (ranging from low to high) and certainty of having an effect (also ranging from low to high), giving a range of outcomes from least (low certainty, low impact) to most (high certainty, high impact). Thus, intensive interventions with small groups or individuals might have high certainty if they consistently result in changes in behaviour but low impact if they result in only a slight improvement on the health status of the community as a whole.

The process for assessing and weighing up potential gains and risks permits a mix of interventions, or a portfolio, to be adopted to balance the risks as a way to maintain health promotion momentum without having complete evidence about the effectiveness of interventions. This approach allows interventions to be selected based on the best available evidence, while not excluding untried but promising strategies.

The investment approach may require different types of information, including costs, likely effectiveness, likely depth and reach of impact, sustainability and acceptability. Further, when investment decisions are made, attention needs to be paid to the effects of upstream policy decisions that affect the context in which prevention policies are implemented.

Core actions

Based on an analysis of the evidence, the recommendations of expert committees, the provisions of internationally agreed strategies and current policy developments in several countries, a set of essential preventive actions can be identified to be part of the proposed action portfolio. Prioritization should be based on national circumstances and level of policy development, but the success of the strategy depends on the simultaneous commitment to macro-level policies and population-wide programmes, regulation and action in the area of nutrition and physical activity. Macro-level policies should always be considered from the viewpoint of their potential effects on low socioeconomic groups.

Actions to promote the demand for and supply of healthy food

1. In **agricultural policy**, agriculture and other aspects of the supply chain should be coherent with public health objectives. The current policy of incentives for sugar and fat production should be revised, in favour of support for the production and marketing of fruit and vegetables. Tariffs restricting trade in fruit and vegetables should be reconsidered. Further, sustainable local production should be encouraged.
2. As to **food composition and product reformulation**, primary producers (such as animal farmers) and food manufacturers should be encouraged and given incentives to revise the characteristics of their products to lower total fat, saturated fat, added sugar and salt.
3. In **food pricing**, economic measures that facilitate healthier food choice and restrict consumption of fats and sugar, such as measures to increase the price of high-energy products and beverages and reduce the price of fruit and vegetables, should be considered, taking into account their effects on low-income groups.
4. In **food distribution and marketing**, urban planners and local governments should consider the location of food outlets. Local markets should be supported and an even distribution of different types of food outlets ensured. Retailers should be encouraged to make more healthy food available in all sales points, at prices affordable for low-income groups. Point-of-sale promotions should be encouraged for healthier options and discouraged for less healthy options.
5. In **catering**, the private sector should be encouraged to provide food choices compatible with food-based dietary guidelines. Takeaway food outlets and lunch bars should be discouraged from promoting energy-dense foods and larger portion sizes through price incentives. The density of food outlets should be considered in the context of urban planning.
6. In **food advertising and promotion**, the volume of commercial promotion of food and non-alcoholic beverages to children should be reduced through both industry self-regulation and statutory action. Promotion should be defined as all forms of communication including competitions, point-of-sale promotion, packaging, contests, sweepstakes, free gifts, product placement, sponsorship, celebrity endorsement, use of cartoon characters, new media such as cell phones and the Internet, and mass media advertising.

7. **Food labelling** should be established to flag products that contain high amounts of fat, sugar, energy and salt. The nutrition labelling scheme should be easily understandable, standardized, and based on an agreed nutrient profiling system.
8. The provision of **foods in schools and kindergartens** should be improved by ensuring that the catering services comply with food-based dietary guidelines, offering fruit and vegetable snacks and cool water and by eliminating energy-dense and nutrient-poor food and beverages from vending machines.
9. In **the workplace**, a variety of food choices compatible with food-based dietary guidelines should be made available. Price incentives and promotion of the healthier options should be provided.
10. Fast-food outlets and vending machines providing energy-dense and nutrient-poor foods should not be located in **hospitals**.
11. As to **information and education**, nutrition education and social marketing campaigns should be regularly performed to encourage the adoption of healthy lifestyles and to inform the public about the health risks of being overweight. A healthy lifestyle culture should be promoted by incorporating positive behaviour change messages in television programmes and in magazines. Nutrition education in schools should be supported.
12. **Food-based dietary guidelines and updated reference nutrient intakes** should be developed with international standardization.
13. As to **breastfeeding and complementary feeding**, support should be given for exclusive breastfeeding by maintaining and expanding baby-friendly hospitals, enforcing the International Code of Marketing of Breast-milk Substitutes, and developing women's labour policies that allow sufficiently long maternity leave and support in the workplace. Guidelines for infant feeding should be provided, as well as training and support to mothers.

Actions to promote physical activity in the population

1. **Health professionals** should provide counselling and give prescriptions in primary care consultations.
2. European transport settings can provide an excellent, though still underexploited opportunity to achieve the recommended daily amount of moderate physical activity for general health benefits. Facilitating the choice of physically **active transport** requires addressing, among others, the safety needs of cyclists and pedestrians, especially children, to promote independent commuting.
3. **Schools and kindergartens** should provide children and adolescents with more and better opportunities for physical activity. To ensure that kindergartens and schools contribute to a considerable part of the recommended daily 60 minutes of varied physical activity for children and young people, a range of different curricular and extracurricular pursuits must be made available.
4. **Urban design and the housing environment** can facilitate or constrain physical activity and active living. The quality of the neighbourhood environment affects residents' opportunities for and willingness to make physically active use of common spaces. Security and safety should be ensured.
5. As to **outdoor recreational activities**, reduced physical exertion in the workplace and home, combined with more leisure time for most people, provides a good basis to increase leisure-time-related physical activity. After decades during which organized sport and specialized sport disciplines have been prioritized through the development and use of facilities, including many expensive and specialized facilities, less active groups must now be made a priority and given increased access to resources to establish an appropriate infrastructure. Opportunities should be created in the local environment that motivate people to engage in physically active leisure. Affordable recreational/exercise facilities, including support for disadvantaged groups, should be offered.
6. The **workplace** should be an ideal setting to promote physical activity to adults. The best results are achieved when specific exercises (training) are performed – preferably designed to complement the amount of physical activity the job entails and individual capacity – at a moderate or vigorous intensity level and on a regular basis, preferably three times a week, with a special focus on the participation of sedentary people. Fiscal measures such as tax breaks for employers should also be considered for improving physical activity.

Actions specific to the health service

1. Diet and lifestyle **counselling** should be provided in primary care to help individuals maintain a healthy weight and to stop the progression from overweight to obesity. Food-based dietary guidelines should be used for this purpose. Higher-risk individuals, such as children of overweight parents, pregnant women, postmenopausal women and individuals undergoing lifestyle changes, should be given special attention and advice. Prescription of physical activity may be considered as an option. Maternity and child health care services should provide specific counselling on diet in pregnancy and on infant and young child feeding.
2. For the **diagnosis and treatment** of obesity co-morbidities, routine anthropometric measurements such as BMI and waist measurements should be carried out at primary care level, in association with screening for associated risk factors (blood pressure, blood lipids, blood glucose). Low-energy diets and increased physical activity are effective in determining a modest total weight loss and in maintaining it. Diet alone appears to be more effective than exercise alone in losing weight. For very obese children or moderately obese children with additional complications, a balanced low-energy diet using normally available foods is recommended. Treating associated health risks and established complications is as important as managing obesity.
3. For the **quality of service delivery**, health ministries and professional organizations should issue clinical recommendations for screening and treatment of obesity. The public sector should ensure that diagnostic practices and dietary prescriptions not supported by the scientific literature are banned.

Actions in training and research

1. Different categories of health staff (in maternity, child, dental, primary, secondary and school health care services) should receive **training** in healthy lifestyles and how to promote them. Health staff should be trained in obesity prevention and management in children and adults. Attention needs to be given to people with coexisting mental disorders and morbid obesity, which require psychological expertise as part of a multidisciplinary approach.
2. Scientists should be involved in **expanding the evidence base** by designing and implementing pilot projects, and by analysing the health impact of policy measures.
3. **Cost–effectiveness analysis** should be applied to ongoing policies, to guide policy-makers' choices.
4. A **monitoring system** observing changes in the level of risk factors and outcome variables should be established and sustained.

Actions should be conducted not only at the national level but also at the regional and local authority levels, and should be tailored to the population's needs and the cultural and regulatory context. Actions should be taken in every age group, but the early life stages, childhood and adolescence, should be emphasized. Legislation should be considered as an important tool for government action.

The role of stakeholders

Within the health sector itself, several actions can be taken to ensure effective population-wide prevention, active prevention in high-risk individuals and optimal delivery of treatment services. Adequate resources will have to be invested in the issue, and the first task will be their identification and mobilization. The use of existing resources will have to be rationalized, to address coherently the issue of obesity across specialities and levels of care. Investment in health promotion through the establishment of community-based interventions and population-wide campaigns on lifestyle change are the primary responsibility of the health sector. Investment is likely to be required in human resources. All categories of staff (doctors, dieticians, nurses) need nutrition training, and primary health care doctors specifically need to have lifestyle counselling skills. Investment in consumables will also be required in primary care settings, so that multiple risk factor assessment is possible. The health sector should guarantee quality standards of service, including by establishing protocols, reducing waiting times and ensuring the availability of services throughout the country, particularly in more deprived areas. The public sector should also ensure that adequate quality of service is given in the private sector, and that inappropriate practices, such as the prescription of dietary advice not supported by the scientific literature, is banned.

Given that the determinants of obesity are wide ranging, many different government departments, extending far beyond health ministries alone, need to be involved in tackling the issue. They include agriculture, education, trade, transport, social welfare, housing and planning, finance, culture, media and sport. The health sector must therefore demonstrate greater capacity in raising awareness of the possible benefits of partnership in order to win the support of other stakeholders. Local governments and communities should be mobilized and supported, and strong networks and alliances built to increase involvement; multisectoral action should be implemented at the local level.

Within the private sector, those concerned extend beyond the food and drink, retail and advertising industries; the construction and design, development, automotive, leisure, media and computer industries can potentially make major contributions. A basic requirement is that all stakeholders agree on their specific roles in the issue. The food and beverage industry should fully acknowledge that it has a role to play in addressing childhood obesity.

Nongovernmental organizations and others in civil society, including professional associations with specialist expertise, consumer organizations and community-focused groups, can all offer valuable policy support and provide access to important knowledge networks and resources that can help to strengthen proposals and reinforce outcomes.

Stakeholder involvement means committing resources to ensure successful, constructive consultation, dialogue or participatory partnerships as part of developing and subsequently implementing public health strategies, especially for prevention. Defining who is a legitimate stakeholder and establishing processes to manage stakeholder involvement are important considerations when determining new approaches to tackling obesity. The process of reconciling the differing stakeholder values of the public and private sectors, as well as nongovernmental organizations and civil-society groups, needs to be carefully managed.

The participation of stakeholders also implies a collaborative or cooperative approach, with a ready consensus on the direction policies should take. Unfortunately, this is rarely the case. As has been shown with tobacco control, governments should be prepared to adopt a parallel approach to strengthen legislative and regulatory measures, as well as adopting novel approaches to achieve maximum benefits from stakeholder participation.

Commercial producers will probably resist attempts to limit their freedom to market products, and strategies should be based on experience in controlling other threats to public health, such as alcohol, tobacco and breast-milk substitutes. Marketing controls may also be justified by invoking the rights of children to an environment free of commercial exploitation. Article 17 of the Convention on the Rights of the Child specifically states that the countries shall "encourage the development of appropriate guidelines for the protection of the child from information and material injurious to his or her well-being" *(140)*.

Monitoring mechanisms are needed to evaluate stakeholder actions: first to estimate how effective they are likely to be, then to monitor delivery and finally to evaluate the effect on obesity or its determinants. The actions envisaged should be assessed to determine whether they will reach a significant proportion of the population or are merely token actions. Experience suggests that rules may be needed for public-sector engagement with the private sector to avoid the appearance that the public sector is endorsing private-sector initiatives – such as providing partial, biased or confusing information – which may not benefit public health and could increase health problems.

Evaluating policy

Monitoring and evaluation are essential components of public health policies and programmes and should be incorporated in every policy measure.

- Outcome indicators need to be clearly defined, standardized between countries, measurable and explicitly linked to public health goals.

- Indicators should be used to measure not only the outcome but also the process and the output of a policy or programme.
- Health impact assessment of policies, with a special focus on obesity, can enhance efforts across the government to counteract obesity, improve the health and well-being of the population and reduce inequality in health. It is a tool for evaluating the health effects of all policies at the national or local level and encourages a multisectoral approach to combating obesity.
- For practical reasons, many obesity studies measure the effect of interventions at a community, local or programme level. The effects of a project or policy at the national level, which deals with the larger social determinants of obesity and the resulting obesogenic environments, are often not assessed. Health impact assessment can be very useful now, since evidence on the impact of policies or programmes at the national level is lacking.
- Obesity urgently needs to be monitored at the local, national and international levels. Data on preschool and primary-school children and specific data on physical activity are deficient.
- The upstream determinants of obesity – such as food availability, pricing, marketing and labelling – need to be monitored at the national and international levels; exposure to these determinants should be monitored according to socioeconomic status.
- The implementation of action needs to be monitored and evaluated and the policies reviewed in the light of the evaluation. Experience suggests that organizations that are independent of commercial and political influence are best able to perform this role. Examples of bodies that could be used to undertake this work include obesity observatories, nutrition councils and public health institutes. Their tasks should include publishing findings and well-structured, publicly accessible reviews undertaken at regular intervals.
- The monitoring bodies need to be independent of political and commercial influence. Their reports should be published regularly.

Policy development: the next steps

Society has to be prepared to accept major changes to its cultural values and aspirations with implications for all aspects of the food chain, social services, leisure activities and wider environmental considerations. Ultimately, personal choice must be effectively expressed, but serious consideration needs to be given to the nature of legislation that will enable this choice to be exercised in a fully informed way and to the rights of individuals, especially children, to health to be fully protected and supported.

Policy interventions to counter obesity that emphasize health education and provide information may have less impact on individuals in households with lower incomes and of lower educational attainment, who lack or perceive that they lack the means to turn the advice into action. In particular, if specific resources – such as money, free time or skills – are needed to improve diet or undertake physical activity, then only the groups with these resources can act on the health education message. Such educational strategies in isolation may therefore only benefit the population groups with better socioeconomic status, thus increasing the differences between them and the more disadvantaged. Health strategies need to include measures to ensure that people with lower socioeconomic status can easily make healthy choices, if they are to avoid widening inequality in health.

The emphasis should be shifted from individual-based to population-based interventions. An ecological approach, acknowledging people's interactions with their physical and sociocultural environments and including influences from different sectors, provides a comprehensive basis for promoting physical activity.

Greater investment in preventing obesity is required. The costs of such intervention can be set against the costs of not intervening: not only the additional health care required for obese individuals but lost productivity, social and family care costs and personal suffering.

European countries are among those at the forefront of developing novel means of promoting increased physical activity through urban design and by providing sports and active leisure facilities, and examples of good practice can be shared through appropriate networks. Similarly, many European governments have a long history of proactive public health policies and good practice in promoting healthy diets and protecting traditional food resources and production methods, and these should be shared and networked.

The capacity to implement policies needs to be reviewed: for example, a lack of sufficient qualified and experienced health care professionals trained in both preventing and managing obesity requires innovative new training programmes based on pan-European standards.

The private sector needs to do more to improve its product portfolios, marketing practices and consumer information. Government incentives for private-sector change include the purchasing power of public-sector catering contracts, which can be used to encourage the production and distribution of healthier food items.

Nongovernmental organizations can be more actively involved in advocating changes in the organizations and institutions responsible for influencing diets and physical activity. Their activities should be supported as part of developing national policy.

Establishing strong, internationally coordinated action to counteract obesity is both a challenge and an opportunity, as many key measures are cross-border in both character and implications.

To address the growing challenge posed by the epidemic of obesity to health, economies and development, the ministers and delegates attending the WHO European Ministerial Conference on Counteracting Obesity (in Istanbul, Turkey, 15–17 November 2006), in the presence of the European Commissioner for Health and Consumer Protection, adopted the European Charter on Counteracting Obesity (Annex 1). The development of the Charter involved different government sectors, international organizations, experts, civil society and the private sector through dialogue and consultations. The Charter is expected to produce a measurable impact in the European Region and beyond, by setting an example and mobilizing global efforts.

References[3]

1. *Obesity: preventing and managing the global epidemic. Report of a WHO Consultation*. Geneva, World Health Organization, 2000 (WHO Technical Report Series, No. 894) (http://www.who.int/nutrition/publications/obesity/en/index.html).
2. Lobstein T, Baur L, Uauy R for the IASO International Obesity Task Force. Obesity in children and young people: a crisis in public health. *Obesity Reviews*, 2004, 5(Suppl. 1):4–104.
3. Cole TJ et al. Establishing a standard definition for child overweight and obesity worldwide: international survey. *British Medical Journal*, 2000, 320:1240–1243.
4. *WHO Child Growth Standards: length/height-for-age, weight-for-age, weight-for-length, weight-for-height, and body mass index-for-age. Methods and development*. Geneva, World Health Organization, 2006 (http://www.who.int/childgrowth/standards/technical_report/en/index.html).
5. WHO Global NCD InfoBase: WHO global comparable estimates [online database]. Geneva, World Health Organization, 2005 (http://www.who.int/ncd_surveillance/infobase/web/InfoBaseCommon).
6. Wang Y, Lobstein T. Worldwide trends in childhood overweight and obesity. *International Journal of Pediatric Obesity*, 2006, 1:11–25.
7. James WPT et al. Overweight and obesity (high body mass index). In: Ezzati M et al., eds. *Comparative quantification of health risks: global and regional burden of disease attribution to selected major risk factors. Vol. 1*. Geneva, World Health Organization, 2004:497–596 (http://www.who.int/publications/cra/en).
8. Yngve A. *Intake of fruit and vegetables in European children and their mothers, folate intake in Swedish children and health indicators – Overweight, plasma homocysteine levels and school performance* [dissertation]. Stockholm, Karolinska University Press, 2005.
9. Currie C et al., eds. *Young people's health in context. Health Behaviour in School-aged Children (HBSC) study: international report from the 2001/2002 survey*. Copenhagen, WHO Regional Office for Europe, 2004 (Health Policy for Children and Adolescents, No. 4) (http://www.euro.who.int/InformationSources/Publications/Catalogue/20040601_1).
10. Elgar FJ et al. Validity of self-reported height and weight and predictors of bias in adolescents. *Journal of Adolescent Health*, 2005, 37:371–375.
11. Baird J et al. Being big or growing fast: systematic review of size and growth in infancy and later obesity. *British Medical Journal*, 2005, 331:929.
12. Johannsson E et al. Tracking of overweight from early childhood to adolescence in cohorts born 1988 and 1994: overweight in a high birth weight population. *International Journal of Obesity*, 2006, 30:1265–1271.
13. Harder T et al. Duration of breastfeeding and risk of overweight: a meta-analysis. *American Journal of Epidemiology*, 2005, 162:397–403.
14. Muenning P et al. Gender and the burden of disease attributable to obesity. *American Journal of Public Health*, 2006, 96(9):1662–1668.
15. Burke JP et al. Impact of case ascertainment on recent trends in diabetes incidence in Rochester, Minnesota. *American Journal of Epidemiology*, 2002, 155(9):859–865.
16. Peeters A et al. Obesity in adulthood and its consequences for life expectancy: a life-table analysis. *Annals of Internal Medicine*, 2003, 138:24–32 (http://www.ajph.org/cgi/content/full/96/9/1662).
17. Department of Health – Economic and Operational Research. *Life expectancy projections, Government Actuary's Department: estimated effect of obesity (based on straight line extrapolation of trends)*. London, The Stationery Office, 2004.

[3] Electronic publications were accessed on 17 January 2007.

18. Dietz WH. Health consequences of obesity in youth: childhood predictors of adult disease. *Pediatrics*, 1998, 101:518–525.
19. Weil E et al. Obesity among adults with disabling conditions. *Journal of the American Medical Association*, 2002, 288:1265–1268.
20. Delvin M et al. Obesity: what mental health professionals need to know. *American Journal of Psychiatry*, 2000:157(6), 854–866.
21. van Hanswijck de Jonge P et al. The prevalence of DSM-IV personality pathology among individuals with bulimia nervosa, binge eating disorder and obesity. *Psychological Medicine*, 2003, 33(7):1311–1317.
22. *Evaluation du coût de l'obésité en Belgique*. Brussels, Institut Belge de l'Economie de la Santé, 2000 (Briefing 29).
23. Thompson D et al. Body mass index and future healthcare costs: a retrospective cohort study. *Obesity Research*, 2001, 9:210–218.
24. Thompson D et al. Lifetime health and economic consequences of obesity. *Archives of Internal Medicine*, 1999, 159:2177–2183.
25. Fry J, Finley W. The prevalence and costs of obesity in the EU. *Proceedings of the Nutrition Society*, 2005, 64(3):359–362.
26. Detournay B et al. Obesity morbidity and health care costs in France: an analysis of the 1991–1992 Medical Care Household Survey. *International Journal of Obesity and Related Metabolic Disorders*, 2000, 24:151–155.
27. Levy E et al. The economic cost of obesity: the French situation. *International Journal of Obesity and Related Metabolic Disorders*, 1995, 19:788–792.
28. Schmid A et al. Economic burden of obesity and its comorbidities in Switzerland. *Soz Praventivmed*, 2005, 50(2):87–94.
29. Polder JJ et al. *Kosten van ziekten in Nederland: de zorgeuro ontrafeld* [Cost of illness in the Netherlands: disentangling the care euro]. Bilthoven, National Institute for Public Health and the Environment, 2002.
30. Polder JJ, Achterberg PW. *Cost of illness in the Netherlands – Highlights*. Bilthoven, National Institute for Public Health and the Environment, 2002.
31. Borg S et al. Obesity, survival and hospital costs – Findings from a screening project in Sweden. *Value in Health*, 2005, 8(5):562–571.
32. House of Commons Health Committee. *Obesity: third report of Session 2003–04. Volume I, report together with formal minutes*. London, The Stationery Office, 2004.
33. *Report on the weight status of NSW: 2003*. Sydney, New South Wales Center for Public Health Nutrition, 2003 (http://www.health.nsw.gov.au/pubs/r/pdf/weight_nut.pdf).
34. Birmingham CL et al. The cost of obesity in Canada. *Canadian Medical Association Journal*, 1999, 160:483–488.
35. Katzmarzyk PT, Janssen I. The economic costs associated with physical inactivity and obesity in Canada: an update. *Canadian Journal of Applied Physiology*, 2004, 29(1):90–115.
36. Kuriyama S et al. Medical care expenditure associated with body mass index in Japan: the Ohsaki Study. *International Journal of Obesity and Related Metabolic Disorders*, 2002, 26:1069–1074.
37. Swinburn B et al. Health care costs of obesity in New Zealand. *International Journal of Obesity and Related Metabolic Disorders*, 1997, 21:891–896.
38. Quesenberry CP Jr et al. Obesity, health services use, and health care costs among members of a health maintenance organization. *Archives of Internal Medicine*, 1998, 158:466–472.
39. Colditz GA. Economic costs of obesity. *American Journal of Clinical Nutrition*, 1992, 55(2):503–507.
40. Wolf AM, Colditz GA. Current estimates of the economic cost of obesity in the United States. *Obesity Research*, 1998, 6:97–106.
41. Finkelstein EA et al. National medical spending attributable to overweight and obesity: how much, and who's paying? *Health Affairs*, 2003 (W3):219–226 (http://content.healthaffairs.org/cgi/reprint/hlthaff.w3.219v1).

42. *The Surgeon General's call to action to prevent and decrease overweight and obesity.* Rockville, MD, US Department of Health and Human Services, 2001 (http://health.utah.gov/obesity/docs/SurgeonGeneralReport.pdf).
43. Suhrcke M et al. *Economic consequences of chronic diseases and the economic rationale for public and private intervention.* London, Oxford Health Alliance, 2005 (http://www.oxha.org/knowledge/publications/05-meeting-documentation/economics_of_chronic_disease_26oct.pdf/view).
44. Monteiro CA et al. Socioeconomic status and obesity in adult populations of developing countries: a review. *Bulletin of the World Health Organization*, 2004, 82:940–946.
45. Sobal J, Stunkard AJ. Socioeconomic status and obesity: a review of the literature. *Psychological Bulletin*, 1989, 105:260–275.
46. Power C. Health and social inequality in Europe. *British Medical Journal*, 1994, 308:1153–1156.
47. Mackenbach JP, Kunst AE. Health and social inequality in Europe. Classification used in paper was misleading [letter]. *British Medical Journal*, 1994, 309:57.
48. Armstrong J et al. Coexistence of social inequalities in undernutrition and obesity in preschool children: population-based cross-sectional study. *Archives of Disease in Childhood*, 2003, 88:671–675.
49. Jotangia D et al. *Obesity among children under 11.* London, National Centre for Social Research, 2005.
50. Walters S, Suhrcke M. *Socioeconomic inequalities in health and health care access in central and eastern Europe and the CIS: a review of the recent literature.* Copenhagen, WHO Regional Office for Europe, 2005 (WHO European Office for Investment for Health and Development Working Paper 2005/1) (http://www.euro.who.int/Document/SED/Socioecon_ineq.pdf).
51. Kuepper-Nybelen J et al. Major differences in prevalence of overweight according to nationality in preschool children living in Germany: determinants and public health implications. *Archives of Disease in Childhood*, 2005, 90:353–363.
52. European Opinion Research Group EEIG. *Eurobarometer: physical activity.* Brussels, European Commission, 2003 (Special Eurobarometer 183-6/Wave 58.2) (http://ec.europa.eu/public_opinion/archives/ebs/ebs_183_6_en.pdf).
53. Elmadfa I, Weichselbaum E, eds. European nutrition and health report 2004. *Annals of Nutrition and Metabolism*, 2004, 48(Suppl. 2).
54. Agudo A et al. Consumption of vegetables, fruit and other plant foods in the European Prospective Investigation into Cancer and Nutrition (EPIC) cohorts from 10 European countries. *Public Health Nutrition*, 2002, 5:1179–1196.
55. Kumanyika S et al. Obesity prevention: the case for action. Public Health Approaches to the Prevention of Obesity (PHAPO) Working Group of the International Obesity Task Force (IOTF). *International Journal of Obesity and Related Metabolic Disorders*, 2002, 26:425–436.
56. Petersen L et al. Longitudinal study of the long-term relation between physical activity and obesity in adults. *International Journal of Obesity and Related Metabolic Disorders*, 2004, 28:105–112.
57. Hill JO, Wyatt HR. Role of physical activity in preventing and treating obesity. *Journal of Applied Physiology*, 2005, 99:765–770.
58. Laaksonen DE et al. Physical activity in the prevention of type 2 diabetes: the Finnish diabetes prevention study. *Diabetes*, 2005, 54:158–165.
59. Bell EA, Rolls BJ. Energy density of foods affects energy intake across multiple levels of fat content in lean and obese women. *American Journal of Clinical Nutrition*, 2001, 73:1010–1018.
60. Stubbs J et al. Energy density of foods: effects on energy intake. *Critical Reviews in Food Science and Nutrition*, 2000, 40:481–515.
61. Howard BV et al. Low-fat dietary pattern and weight change over 7 years. The women's health initiative dietary modification trial. *Journal of the American Medical Association*, 2006, 295(1):39–49.
62. Howarth NC et al. Dietary fibre and weight regulation. *Nutrition Reviews*, 2001, 59:129–139.

63. Mattes RD, Rothacker D. Beverage viscosity is inversely related to postprandial hunger in humans. *Physiology & Behavior*, 2001, 74:551–557.
64. Pereira MA et al. Fast-food habits, weight gain, and insulin resistance (the CARDIA study): 15-year prospective analysis. *Lancet*, 2005, 365:36–42.
65. Ledikwe JH et al. Portion sizes and the obesity epidemic. *Journal of Nutrition*, 2005, 135:905–909.
66. He K et al. Changes in intake of fruits and vegetables in relation to risk of obesity and weight gain among middle-aged women. *International Journal of Obesity*, 2004, 28:1569–1574.
67. Schulz M et al. Food groups as predictors for short-term weight changes in men and women of the EPIC-Potsdam cohort. *Journal of Nutrition*, 2002, 132:1335–1340.
68. Tooze JA et al. Psychosocial predictors of energy underreporting in a large doubly labeled water study. *American Journal of Clinical Nutrition*, 2004, 79:795–804.
69. *Framework for alcohol policy in the WHO European Region*. Copenhagen, WHO Regional Office for Europe, 2006 (http://www.euro.who.int/document/e88335.pdf).
70. Harrington KE et al. Macronutrient intakes and food sources in Irish adults: findings of the North/South Ireland Food Consumption Survey. *Public Health Nutrition*, 2001, 4:1051–1060.
71. *Zo eet Nederland 1998: resultaten van de Voedselconsumptiepeiling 1998* [This is how the Netherlands eats in 1998: results of the 1998 food consumption survey]. The Hague, Netherlands Nutrition Centre, 1998.
72. De Vriese SR, et al. Enquête de consommation alimentaire Belge 1 – 2004 [web site]. Brussels, Scientific Institute of Public Health, 2006 (http://www.iph.fgov.be/epidemio/epifr/foodfr/table04.htm).
73. DAFNE data food networking. The Pan-European Food Data Bank based on household budget surveys [online database]. Athens, National and Kapodistrian University of Athens, 2005 (http://www.nut.uoa.gr/dafnesoftweb).
74. French SA. Public health strategies for dietary change: schools and workplaces. *Journal of Nutrition*, 2005, 135:910–912.
75. *Diet, nutrition and the prevention of chronic diseases. Report of the joint WHO/FAO expert consultation.* Geneva, World Health Organization, 2003 (WHO Technical Report Series No. 916) (http://www.who.int/dietphysicalactivity/publications/trs916/download/en/index.html).
76. *Marketing of food and non-alcoholic beverages to children. Report of a WHO Forum and Technical Meeting, Oslo, Norway, 2–5 May 2006*. Geneva, World Health Organization, 2006 (http://www.who.int/dietphysicalactivity/publications/Oslo%20meeting%20layout%2027%20NOVEMBER.pdf).
77. Hastings G et al. *Review of research on the effects of food promotion to children. Final report*. Glasgow, Centre for Social Marketing, 2003 (http://www.ism.stir.ac.uk/projects_food.htm).
78. McGinnis JM et al. *Food marketing to children and youth: threat or opportunity?* Washington, DC, National Academies Press, 2006.
79. Lobstein T, Dibb S. Evidence of a possible link between obesogenic food advertising and child overweight. *Obesity Reviews*, 2005, 6:203–208.
80. Dowler E. Inequalities in diet and physical activity in Europe. *Public Health Nutrition*, 2001, 4:701–709.
81. Pickett KE et al. Wider income gaps, wider waistbands? An ecological study of obesity and income inequality. *Journal of Epidemiology and Community Health*, 2005, 59:670–674.
82. Finkelstein E et al. Economic causes and consequences of obesity. *Annual Review of Public Health*, 2005, 26:239–257.
83. Carpenter K et al. Relationships between obesity and DSM-IV major depressive disorder, suicide ideation, and suicide attempts: results from a general population study. *American Journal of Public Health*, 2000, 90:251–257.
84. Allison DB et al. The impact of weight gain on quality of life among persons with schizophrenia. *Psychiatric Services*, 2003, 54(4):565–567.
85. Faulkner G et al. Schizophrenia and weight management: a systematic review of interventions to control weight. *Acta Psychiatrica Scandinavica*, 2003, 108(5):324–332.

86. Meyer JM. Awareness of obesity and weight issues among chronically mentally ill inpatients: a pilot study. *Annals of Clinical Psychiatry*, 2002, 14(1):39–45.
87. Antipsychotic-induced weight gain and metabolic abnormalities: implications for increased mortality in patients with schizophrenia. *Journal of Clinical Psychiatry*, 2004, 65(Suppl. 7):4–18.
88. Allison DB et al. Antipsychotic-induced weight gain: a comprehensive research synthesis. *American Journal of Psychiatry*, 1999, 156:1686–1696.
89. Hill AJ, Williams J. Psychological health in a non-clinical sample of obese women. *International Journal of Obesity*, 1998, 22(6):578–583.
90. French SA et al. Self-esteem and obesity in children and adolescents: a literature review. *Obesity Research*, 1995, 3:479–490.
91. Falkner NH et al. Social, educational, and psychological correlates of weight status in adolescents. *Obesity Research*, 2001, 9:32–42.
92. McElroy SL et al. Are mood disorders and obesity related? A review for the mental health professional. *Journal of Clinical Psychiatry*, 2004, 65(5):634–651.
93. Summerbell C et al. *A systematic review of the effectiveness of interventions, including family interventions (in children aged 5–12), to prevent excess weight gain or maintain a healthy weight in children aged between two and five years*. Middlesborough, University of Teesside, 2005.
94. Tedstone A et al. *Effectiveness of interventions to promote healthy eating in preschool children aged 1 to 5 years: a review*. London, Health Education Authority, 1998.
95. Jackson Y et al. Summary of the 2000 Surgeon General's listening session: toward a national action plan on overweight and obesity. *Obesity Research*, 2002, 10(12):1299–1305.
96. Katz DL et al. Public health strategies for preventing and controlling overweight and obesity in school and worksite settings: a report on recommendations of the Task Force on Community Preventive Services. *Mortality and Morbidity Weekly Report*, 2005, 54:1–11.
97. Aldana SG et al. Financial impact of health promotion programs: a comprehensive review of the literature. *American Journal of Health Promotion*, 2001, 15(5):296–320.
98. Lowe CF et al. Effects of a peer modelling and rewards-based intervention to increase fruit and vegetable consumption in children. *European Journal of Clinical Nutrition*, 2004, 58:510–522.
99. Damon S et al. PRESTO – Prevention study of obesity: a project to prevent obesity during childhood and adolescence. *Acta Paediatrica*, 2005, 94(Suppl. 448):47–48.
100. Mamalakis G et al. Obesity indices in a cohort of primary school children in Crete: a six year prospective study. *International Journal of Obesity*, 2000, 24:765–771.
101. Manios Y et al. Health and nutrition education in primary schools of Crete: changes in chronic disease risk factors following a 6-year intervention programme. *British Journal of Nutrition*, 2002, 88:315–324.
102. Nielsen J, Gerlow J. *Evaluering af projekt for familier med overvægtige børn* [Evaluation of a project for families with overweight children]. Copenhagen, Udviklings- og Formidlingscenter for Børn og Unge, 2004.
103. Muller MJ et al. Prevention of obesity – More than an intention. Concept and first results of Kiel Obesity Prevention Study (KOPS). *International Journal of Obesity*, 2001, 25(1):66–74.
104. Graf C et al. Data from the StEP TWO programme showing the effect on blood pressure and different parameters for obesity in overweight and obese primary school children. *Cardiology in the Young*, 2005, 15:291–298.
105. Eliakim A et al. The effect of a combined intervention on body mass index and fitness in obese children and adolescents – A clinical experience. *European Journal of Pediatrics*, 2002, 161:449–454.
106. Warren JM et al. Evaluation of a pilot school programme aimed at the prevention of obesity in children. *Health Promotion International*, 2003, 18:287–296.
107. Reilly JJ, McDowell ZC. Physical activity interventions in the prevention and treatment of paediatric obesity: systematic review and critical appraisal. *Proceedings of the Nutrition Society*, 2003, 62:611–619.

108. Sahota P et al. Evaluation of implementation and effect of primary school based intervention to reduce risk factors for obesity. *British Medical Journal*, 2001, 323:1027–1029.
109. Sahota P et al. Randomised controlled trial of primary school based intervention to reduce risk factors for obesity. *British Medical Journal*, 2001, 323:1029–1032.
110. Kahn EB et al. The effectiveness of interventions to increase physical activity. A systematic review. *American Journal of Preventive Medicine*, 2002, 22(4 Suppl 1):73–107.
111. Guo X et al. Food price policy can favorably alter macronutrient intake in China. *Journal of Nutrition*, 1999, 129:994–1001.
112. Palmer D. *Expanding waistlines/contracting multiples?* Warburg, UBS Investment Research, 2005.
113. *Ottawa Charter for Health Promotion*. Copenhagen, WHO Regional Office for Europe, 1986 (http://www.euro.who.int/AboutWHO/Policy/20010827_2).
114. *The Bangkok Charter for Health Promotion in a Globalized World*. Geneva, World Health Organization, 2005 (http://www.who.int/healthpromotion/conferences/6gchp/bangkok_charter/en/index.html).
115. Smed S et al. Differentiated food taxes as a tool in health and nutrition policy. *XIth International Congress of the European Association of Agricultural Economists, Copenhagen, Denmark, 24–27 August 2005* (http://www.eaae2005.dk/CONTRIBUTED_PAPERS/S23_474_Jensen&Smed.pdf).
116. *Fruit and vegetable promotion initiative: a meeting report, 25–27/08/03*. Geneva, World Health Organization, 2003 (WHO/NMH/NPH/NNP/0308) (http://www.who.int/dietphysicalactivity/publications/f&v_promotion_initiative_report.pdf).
117. Aimbetova G. A health boost for school children. *Network News: European Network of Health Promoting Schools*, 2002, 7:50 (http://www.euro.who.int/document/enhps/ENHPSnews072002.pdf).
118. Case study of Norway. In: *UK law: briefing paper*. Cambridge, Baby Milk Action, 1997 (http://www.babymilkaction.org/pages/uklaw.html#1).
119. *Urban and Peri-urban Food and Nutrition Action Plan: elements for community action to promote social cohesion and reduce inequalities through local production for local consumption*. Copenhagen, WHO Regional Office for Europe, 2001 (http://www.euro.who.int/document/e72949.pdf).
120. Carr S. Water in school is cool! *Health News for Schools*, 2004, 16:2 (http://www.beh.nhs.uk/healthwise/pdf/Schlnews16.pdf).
121. What is a walking bus [web site]? Welwyn Garden City, Mouchel Parkman Services, 2003 (http://www.walkingbus.com).
122. Wardle J et al. Mass education for obesity prevention: the penetration of the BBC's "Fighting Fat, Fighting Fit" campaign. *Health Education Research*, 2001, 16:343–355.
123. *Guidance on the use of sibutramine for the treatment of obesity in adults*. London, National Institute for Clinical Excellence, 2001 (Technology Appraisal Guidance No.31).
124. *Guidance on the use of orlistat for the treatment of obesity in adults*. London, National Institute for Clinical Excellence, 2001 (Technology Appraisal Guidance No.22).
125. Loh C et al. A comprehensive review of behavioural interventions for weight management in schizophrenia. *Annals of Clinical Psychiatry*, 2006, 18(1):23–31.
126. Umbricht D et al. Cognitive behaviour therapy for weight gain. *American Journal of Psychiatry*, 2001, 158:971.
127. Merriman S et al. Wonderful me!: Evaluation of multidisciplinary therapy package for overweight psychiatric patients. *British Journal of Therapy and Rehabilitation*, 1995, 2(10):531–535.
128. Bogers RP et al. *Costs of lifestyle interventions within healthcare and the amount of weight loss achieved*. Bilthoven, National Institute for Public Health and the Environment, 2006 (RIVM Report 260701002/2006).
129. WHO Global Strategy on Diet, Physical Activity and Health [web site]. Geneva, World Health Organization, 2006 (http://www.who.int/dietphysicalactivity/en).

130. Physical Activity and Health – EU Platform for Action [web site]. Brussels, European Commission, 2006 (http://ec.europa.eu/health/ph_determinants/life_style/nutrition/platform/platform_en.htm).
131. Gaining health. *The European Strategy for the Prevention and Control of Noncommunicable Diseases.* Copenhagen, WHO Regional Office for Europe, 2006 (http://www.euro.who.int/InformationSources/Publications/Catalogue/20061003_1).
132. *Global Strategy for Infant and Young Child Feeding.* Geneva, World Health Organization, 2003 (http://www.who.int/child-adolescent-health/New_Publications/NUTRITION/gs_iycf.pdf).
133. Nutrition policy [web site]. Brussels, European Commission, 2006 (http://europa.eu.int/comm/health/ph_determinants/life_style/nutrition/nutrition_policy_en.htm).
134. *European strategy for child and adolescent health and development.* Copenhagen, WHO Regional Office for Europe, 2005 (http://www.euro.who.int/document/E87710.pdf).
135. Children's Environment and Health Action Plan for Europe [web site]. Copenhagen, WHO Regional Office for Europe, 2004 (http://www.euro.who.int/childhealthenv/policy/20020724_2).
136. Pan-European programme on transport, health and environment [web site]. Copenhagen, WHO Regional Office for Europe, 2006 (http://www.euro.who.int/transport/policy/20021009_1).
137. *Nutrition, physical activity and prevention of obesity: recent policy developments in the WHO European Region.* Copenhagen, WHO Regional Office for Europe, 2006 (http://www.euro.who.int/Document/NUT/Instanbul_conf_ebd01.pdf).
138. Hawe P, Shiell A. Preserving innovation under increasing accountability pressures: the health promotion investment portfolio approach. *Health Promotion Journal of Australia*, 1995, 5:4–9.
139. Swinburn B et al. Obesity prevention: a proposed framework for translating evidence into action. *Obesity Reviews*, 2005, 6:23–33.
140. *Convention on the Rights of the Child.* New York, United Nations, 1989 (http://www.unhchr.ch/html/menu3/b/k2crc.htm).

Annex 1. European Charter on Counteracting Obesity

To address the growing challenge posed by the epidemic of obesity to health, economies and development, we, the Ministers and delegates attending the WHO European Ministerial Conference on Counteracting Obesity (Istanbul, Turkey, 15–17 November 2006), in the presence of the European Commissioner for Health and Consumer Protection, hereby adopt, as a matter of policy, the following European Charter on Counteracting Obesity. The process of developing the present Charter has involved different government sectors, international organizations, experts, civil society and the private sector through dialogue and consultations.

We declare our commitment to strengthen action on counteracting obesity in line with this Charter and to place this issue high on the political agenda of our governments. We also call on all partners and stakeholders to take stronger action against obesity and we recognize the leadership on this issue being provided by the WHO Regional Office for Europe.

Sufficient evidence exists for immediate action; at the same time, the search for innovation, adjustments to local circumstances and new research on certain aspects can improve the effectiveness of policies.

Obesity is a global public health problem; we acknowledge the role that European action can play in setting an example and thereby mobilizing global efforts.

1. The challenge

We acknowledge that:

1.1 **The epidemic of obesity poses one of the most serious public health challenges in the WHO European Region**. The prevalence of obesity has risen up to three-fold in the last two decades. Half of all adults and one in five children in the WHO European Region are overweight. Of these, one third are already obese, and numbers are increasing fast. Overweight and obesity contribute to a large proportion of noncommunicable diseases, shortening life expectancy and adversely affecting the quality of life. More than one million deaths in the Region annually are due to diseases related to excess body weight.

1.2 **The trend is particularly alarming in children and adolescents**, thus passing the epidemic into adulthood and creating a growing health burden for the next generation. The annual rate of increase in the prevalence of childhood obesity has been rising steadily and is currently up to ten times higher than it was in 1970.

1.3 **Obesity also strongly affects economic and social development**. Adult obesity and overweight are responsible for up to 6% of health care expenditure in the European Region; in addition, they impose indirect costs (due to the loss of lives, productivity and related income) that are at least two times higher. Overweight and obesity most affect people in lower socioeconomic groups, and this in turn contributes to a widening of health and other inequalities.

1.4 **The epidemic has built up in recent decades as a result of the changing social, economic, cultural and physical environment**. An energy imbalance in the population has been triggered by a dramatic reduction of physical activity and changing dietary patterns, including increased consumption of energy-dense nutrient-poor food and beverages (containing high proportions of saturated as well as total fat, salt, and sugars) in combination with insufficient consumption of fruit and vegetables. According to available data two thirds of the adult population in most countries in the WHO European Region are not physically active enough to secure and maintain health gains, and only in a few countries does the consumption of fruit and vegetables achieve the recommended levels. Genetic predisposition alone can not explain the epidemic of obesity without such changes in the social, economic, cultural and physical environment.

1.5 International action is essential to support national policies. Obesity is no longer a syndrome of wealthy societies; it is becoming just as dominant in developing countries and countries with economies in transition, particularly in the context of globalization. Taking intersectoral action remains a challenge, and no country has yet effectively managed to bring the epidemic under control. Establishing strong internationally coordinated action to counteract obesity is both a challenge and an opportunity, as many key measures are cross-border both in character and in their implications.

2. What can be done: the goals, principles and framework for action

2.1 The obesity epidemic is reversible. It is possible to reverse the trend and bring the epidemic under control. This can only be done by comprehensive action, since the root of the problem lies in the rapidly changing social, economic and environmental determinants of people's lifestyles. The vision is to shape societies where healthy lifestyles related to diet and physical activity are the norm, where health goals are aligned with those related to the economy, society and culture and where healthy choices are made more accessible and easy for individuals.

2.2 Curbing the epidemic and reversing the trend are the ultimate goal of action in the Region. Visible progress, especially relating to children and adolescents, should be achievable in most countries in the next 4–5 years and it should be possible to reverse the trend by 2015 at the latest.

2.3 The following principles need to guide action in the WHO European Region:

2.3.1 High-level political will and leadership and whole-government commitment are required to achieve mobilization and synergies across different sectors.

2.3.2 Action against obesity should be linked to overall strategies to address noncommunicable diseases and health promotion activities, as well as to the broader context of sustainable development. Improved diet and physical activity will have a substantial and often rapid impact on public health, beyond the benefits related to reducing overweight and obesity.

2.3.3 A balance must be struck between the responsibility of individuals and that of government and society. Holding individuals alone accountable for their obesity should not be acceptable.

2.3.4 It is essential to set the action taken within the cultural context of each country or region and to acknowledge the pleasure afforded by a healthy diet and physical activity.

2.3.5 It will be essential to build partnerships between all stakeholders such as government, civil society, the private sector, professional networks, the media and international organizations, across all levels (national, sub-national and local).

2.3.6 Policy measures should be coordinated in the different parts of the Region, in particular to avoid shifting the market pressure for energy-dense food and beverages to countries with less regulated environments. WHO can play a role in facilitating and supporting intergovernmental coordination.

2.3.7 Special attention needs to be focused on vulnerable groups such as children and adolescents, whose inexperience or credulity should not be exploited by commercial activities.

2.3.8 It is also a high priority to support lower socioeconomic population groups, who face more constraints and limitations on making healthy choices. Increasing the access to and affordability of healthy choices should therefore be a key objective.

2.3.9 Impact on public health objectives should have priority consideration when developing economic policy, as well as policies in the areas of trade, agriculture, transport and urban planning.

2.4 A framework, linking the main actors, policy tools and settings, is needed to translate these principles into action.

2.4.1 **All relevant government sectors and levels should play a role.** Appropriate institutional mechanisms need to be in place to enable this collaboration.

- Health ministries should play a leading role by advocating, inspiring and guiding multisectoral action. They should set the example when facilitating healthy choices among employees in the health sector and health service users. The role of the health system is also important when dealing with people at high risk and those already overweight and obese, by designing and promoting prevention measures and by providing diagnosis, screening and treatment.
- All relevant ministries and agencies such as those for agriculture, food, finance, trade and economy, consumer affairs, development, transport, urban planning, education and research, social welfare, labour, sport, culture and tourism have an essential role to play in developing health promoting policies and actions. This will also lead to benefits in their own domain.
- Local authorities have great potential and a major role to play in creating the environment and opportunities for physical activity, active living and a healthy diet, and they should be supported in doing this.

2.4.2 **Civil society can support the policy response.** The active involvement of civil society is important, to foster the public's awareness and demand for action and as a source of innovative approaches. Nongovernmental organizations can support strategies to counteract obesity. Employers', consumers', parents', youth, sport and other associations and trade unions can each play a specific role. Health professionals' organizations should ensure that their members are fully engaged in preventive action.

2.4.3 **The private sector should play an important role and have responsibility in building a healthier environment, as well as for promoting healthy choices in their own workplace.** This includes enterprises in the entire food chain from primary producers to retailers. Action should be focused on the main domain of their activities, such as manufacturing, marketing and product information, while consumer education could also play a role, within the framework set by public health policy. There is also an important role for sectors such as sports clubs, leisure and construction companies, advertisers, public transportation, active tourism, etc. The private sector could be involved in win–win solutions by highlighting the economic opportunities of investing in healthier options.

2.4.4 **The media have an important responsibility** to provide information and education, raise awareness and support public health policies in this area.

2.4.5 **Intersectoral collaboration is essential not only at national but also at international level.** WHO should inspire, coordinate and lead the international action. International organizations such as the United Nations Food and Agriculture Organization (FAO), the United Nations Children's Fund (UNICEF), the World Bank, the Council of Europe, the International Labour Organization (ILO), and the Organisation for Economic Co-operation and Development (OECD) can create effective partnerships and thus stimulate multisectoral collaboration at national and international levels. The European Union (EU) has a principal role to play through EU legislation, public health policy and programmes, research and activities such as the European Platform for Action on Diet, Physical Activity and Health.

Existing international commitments such as the Global Strategy on Diet, Physical Activity and Health, the European Food and Nutrition Action Plan and the European Strategy for the Prevention and Control of Noncommunicable Diseases should be used for guidance and to create synergies. In addition, policy commitments such as the Children's Environment and Health Action Programme for Europe (CEHAPE), the Transport, Health and Environment Pan-European Programme (THE PEP), and the Codex Alimentarius within the limits of its remit, can be used to achieve coherence and consistency in international action and to maximize efficient use of resources.

2.4.6 **Policy tools range from legislation to public/private partnerships, with particular importance attached to regulatory measures.** Government and national parliaments should ensure consistency and sustainability through regulatory action, including legislation. Other important tools include policy reformulation, fiscal and public investment policies, health impact assessment, campaigns to raise awareness and provide consumer information, capacity building and partnership, research, planning and monitoring. Public/private partnerships with a public health rationale and shared specified public health objectives should be encouraged. Specific regulatory measures should include: the adoption of regulations to substantially reduce the extent and impact of commercial promotion of energy-dense foods and beverages, particularly to children, with the development of international approaches, such as a code on marketing to children in this area; and the adoption of regulations for safer roads to promote cycling and walking.

2.4.7 **Action should be taken at both micro and macro levels, and in different settings.** Particular importance is attached to settings such as the home and families, communities, kindergartens, schools, workplaces, means of transport, the urban environment, housing, health and social services, and leisure facilities. Action should also cover the local, country and international levels. Through this, individuals should be supported and encouraged to take responsibility by actively using the possibilities offered.

2.4.8 **Action should be aimed at ensuring an optimal energy balance by stimulating a healthier diet and physical activity.** While information and education will remain important, the focus should shift to a portfolio of interventions designed to change the social, economic and physical environment to favour healthy lifestyles.

2.4.9 **A package of essential preventive actions should be promoted as key measures; countries may further prioritize interventions from this package, depending on their national circumstances and the level of policy development.** The package of essential action would include: reduction of marketing pressure, particularly to children; promotion of breastfeeding; ensuring access to and availability of healthier food, including fruit and vegetables; economic measures that facilitate healthier food choices; offers of affordable recreational/exercise facilities, including support for socially disadvantaged groups; reduction of fat, free (particularly added) sugars and salt in manufactured products; adequate nutrition labelling; promotion of cycling and walking by better urban design and transport policies; creation of opportunities in local environments that motivate people to engage in leisure time physical activity; provision of healthier foods, opportunities for daily physical activity, and nutrition and physical education in schools; facilitating and motivating people to adopt better diets and physical activity in the workplace; developing/improving national food-based dietary guidelines and guidelines for physical activity; and individually adapted health behaviour change.

2.4.10 **Attention should also continue to be focused on preventing obesity in people who are already overweight and thus at high risk, and on treating the disease of obesity.** Specific actions in this area would include: introducing timely identification and management of overweight and obesity in primary care, provision of training for health professionals in the prevention of obesity; and issuing clinical guidance for screening and treatment. Any stigmatization or overvaluation of obese people should be avoided at any age.

2.4.11 **When designing and implementing policies, successful interventions with demonstrated effectiveness need to be used.** These include projects with proven impact on the consumption of healthier foods and levels of physical activity such as: schemes to offer people free fruit at school; affordable pricing for healthier foods; increasing access to healthier foods at workplaces and in areas of socioeconomic deprivation; establishing bicycle priority routes; encouraging children to walk to school; improving street lighting; promoting stair use; and reducing television viewing. There is also evidence that many interventions against obesity, such as school programmes and active transport, are highly cost-effective. The WHO Regional Office for Europe will provide decision-makers with examples of good practice and case studies.

3. Progress and monitoring

3.1 The present Charter aims to strengthen action against obesity throughout the WHO European Region. It will stimulate and influence national policies, regulatory action including legislation and action plans. A European action plan, covering nutrition and physical activity, will translate the principles and framework provided by the Charter into specific action packages and monitoring mechanisms.

3.2 A process needs to be put together to develop internationally comparable core indicators for inclusion in national health surveillance systems. These data could then be used for advocacy, policy-making and monitoring purposes. This would also allow for regular evaluation and review of policies and actions and for the dissemination of findings to a wide audience.

3.3 Monitoring progress on a long-term basis is essential, as the outcomes in terms of reduced obesity and the related disease burden will take time to manifest themselves. Three-year progress reports should be prepared at the WHO European level, with the first due in 2010.

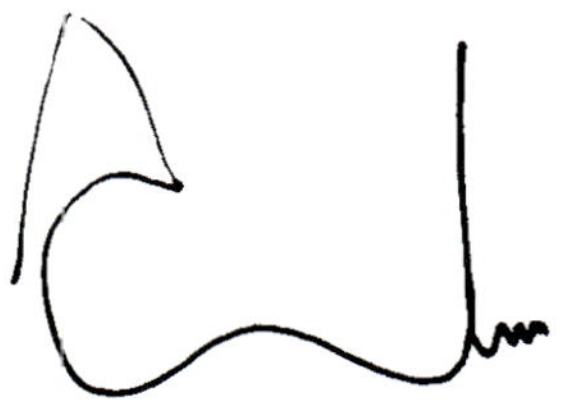

Professor Recep Akdağ
Minister of Health of Turkey

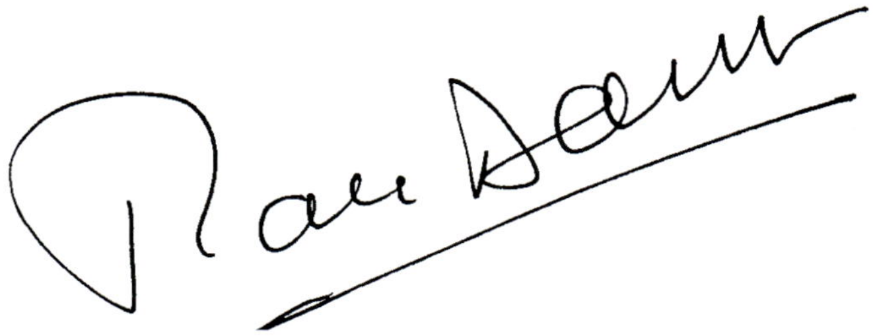

Dr Marc Danzon
WHO Regional Director for Europe

Istanbul, 16 November 2006